EMOTIONAL INTELLIGENCE & CRITICAL THINKING SKILLS FOR LEADERSHIP (2 IN 1)

20 MUST KNOW STRATEGIES TO BOOST YOUR EQ, IMPROVE YOUR SOCIAL SKILLS & SELF-AWARENESS AND BECOME A BETTER LEADER

STEWART HUNTER

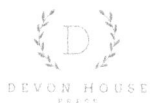

DEVON HOUSE
PRESS

CONTENTS

Part V

BUILDING BETTER RELATIONSHIPS,
THRIVING IN YOUR CHOSEN PATH, &
BECOMING THE BEST LEADER THAT YOU
CAN BE

INTRODUCTION

Leadership. It's a prized position, a measure of personal and professional respect. Many strive for it but few achieve it. Some believe it's inborn into a person's personality, that only the naturally charismatic can be true leaders. Others may feel their leadership waning, control over professional and personal aspects of their lives slipping away. Their leadership skills need improving and fast, before it's too late.

Whatever your specific situation, you're reading this now because you want to strengthen your leadership skills, if that's possible. And, of course, it is. Any skillset can be sharpened, and leadership skills are crucial to so many aspects of life; personal, professional, social, familial. The better your leadership skills, the better your life will be and the happier and more fulfilled you and those around you will be.

And this book has the answers you need! You'll learn everything you need to know and more about psychological principles and research-based concepts which are backed up with easy-to-use tests you can take on the spot. We break down leadership skills like clear communication, empathy, reflection (among many others) and what they entail; emotional intelligence, cognitive abilities, critical thinking, and social skills. We'll apply these skills to various arenas and stages of life, demonstrating how certain basic concepts are consistent in any type of development. The latest medical information and industry data is compiled in this easy-to-read handbook for leadership self-improvement.

We publish books designed to improve every part of your personal and professional life, with a staff of dedicated writers and researchers to help you overcome your challenges, achieve your goals, and have a happier, longer, and more fulfilling life. I've personally used these techniques myself and I can vouch for their efficacy. They will make you more emotionally intelligent, more self-aware, more mindful and grateful, more relaxed and stress free. Even a small handful of the principles in this book could turn any life or career around. Using all of them could be revolutionary for you and anyone you know or love.

This book has all you need to get started right away, from home or the office or where ever you are. In fact, if you are paying attention, ready to focus, retain, recall, and apply this information, you've already taken the first step to better leadership skills. Now turn the page and take the next step. The time is now. If you're finally reading this, then you've been thinking about this for a while. There could be problems in your workplace or home even now, and they're likely getting worse. Miscommunication, disorganization, disrespect, and dissatisfaction can (and will) fester in silence, they grow in the shadows. Things in your marriage or career or with your kids or friends or adult siblings could already be approaching a crisis point. Or you may go on languishing on the lower rungs of life for another month, another year, another decade.

Time is the one thing money can't buy, the only thing we cannot afford to waste. So, don't waste another second! Start improving your life now, while there's still time!

Heightened emotional intelligence, sharper cognitive and critical thinking skills, the keys to repairing or creating stronger relationships and superior team results are in your hands, yours for the taking. Enjoy the journey and don't worry, you won't be alone. Now let's move forward to a better career and a better life!

I

SELF-CHECK: WHAT KIND OF LEADER ARE YOU RIGHT NOW?

ARE YOU A TRUE LEADER?

We can vaguely define *leadership* as the process of influencing others to accomplish some objective by means of coherent and cohesive organization. But that's a lot easier said than done. What makes a good leader? Are you one, or is there room for improvement? Do you have what it takes to be the leader you aspire to be? The answer, of course, is yes, or we wouldn't have published this book. It's a handy guide to make you the leader you want and need to be.

But what kind of leader is that?

A LEADER IN NAME ONLY

You're a leader, a true leader. Your concern is the efficiency of your staff and the accuracy and efficacy of the results. You know your workers are crucial and you value their humanity as well as their utility. You and your team can be trusted to get the job done. Otherwise, what kind of leader are you?

Sadly, you'd be like most in that position, a leader in name only. This is an easier trap to fall into, and most people who do it don't even realize. It may even have happened to you, despite your best efforts to the contrary.

Scary, right? You could be asleep at the wheel without even knowing it. But it's never too late to snap out of it and take control of your team again. Ask yourself some of these helpful questions to make sure you're not a leader in name only.

What's really more important to you, the results of the project or the benefit to your career? Be honest. A lot of people put their career first because we're trained to do that. Our competitive society, especially in the United States, gears us to base our entire identities on what we do, how much we earn. Status symbols are everywhere, from the cars we drive to the houses we live in. Our success is often the measure of our worth, the measure of our humanity. Furthermore, a person's career will have a lot of projects, just as a doctor's career will have a lot of patients and an accountant's career a lot of taxpayers. What matters more to the accountant or doctor or manager? A doctor may lose a patient, but he or she still has a house to pay for, kids to feed, clothe, and put through school. An accountant has clients who come and go, but only one family, one career to see to that family.

So, it's common and it's not unreasonable. But it's not good leadership. Because a good leader understands that the ultimate success of that singular career is based on the successes of the smaller units, the project or the patient or the taxpayer. Too many losses or failures and the doctor or accountant's careers dry up. Even if the patients and taxpayers keep coming (and they will) there's a matter of professional integrity. The good doctor or accountant does a good job for their patient or taxpayer, they do the best they can do every time. Sometimes mistakes are made, and they can often be corrected. But a leader knows that he or she is not the center of the project. A good doctor doesn't go into the operating room concerned with their reputation; they go in concerned for their patient. The accountant may know he or she will have to stand behind their work, but first and foremost they should be concerned with the accuracy of the tax return they're creating. That's the measure of their professional worth.

It brings us to an important concept, one you must know. Successful people prioritize the end result and not their place in the project. It's a sign of security and self-actualization to put the project above the person. It's an externalizing technique which separates the person from the behavior which allows failures to be seen as stepping stones to success instead of as stains on a person's reputation. Too many failures will have an adverse effect professionally, of course, but that can lead to overthinking and negative self-talk, and they can put anyone, manager or worker, into a destructive downward spiral.

Overthinking, in brief, is the tendency to endlessly ponder what could have been done in the past, or what might be done in the future. Replaying old arguments while inserting rewritten lines or imagining conversations which have yet to occur (and may never) are good ways to waste time and energy and generate anxiety and stress.

Negative self-talk is the tendency to tell one's self that they're worthless, doomed to failure. It's the self-punishment that goes along with overthinking, and it's absolutely toxic. No good leader indulges in this harmful practice.

It comes down to a mindset; either a fixed mindset or a growth mindset. A fixed mindset associates the person with the events around them, the way a leader in name only may do. The fixed mindset believes the results are foretold, because if a person had had a failure, they must be a failure, and they always will be a failure. Overthinking and negative self-talk help to ensure this mindset, and it influences behavior. Lack of self-confidence will either restrict opportunities or create failures through the principle of the self-fulfilling prophecy.

A growth mindset accepts failure as a learning experience and is necessary to ultimate success. This mindset externalizes the events from the person, they believe a person may fail without being a failure, that they can grow through the process of failures. This mindset tends to avoid overthinking about the past or future and focuses more on the present, on getting the job done. They indulge in positive self-talk, supporting themselves with self-sympathy. This gives them the confidence to take on new opportunities and have new successes because of the principle of the self-fulfilling prophecy.

The leader in name only is likely to have a fixed mindset. The true leader is likely to have a growth mindset. Which mindset do you have? Are you a true leader or a leader in name only?

Are you consistent? We mentioned integrity before, and it's time to take a closer look at that. It's an aeronautical term, referring to the wing of a plane. The wing is expected to bend and yield to certain external forces like wind and temperature. But integrity refers to the way in which the wing responds. Given the same external forces, the wing should react in a predictable, reliable fashion. That is known as the integrity of the wing. When this integrity is violated and the wing is reacting in an unreliable, unstable manner, it may tear off and cause the plane to crash.

People are the same way. They react to the forces around them, a supervisor or a puppy dog elicit different reactions. But a person should generally be reliable in their reaction to each. And a wing is still a wing, it doesn't act like an engine or a window. It is what it is and does what it does no matter what the elevation, if the plane is moving or not. People likewise shouldn't become radically different people in one person's company or another. Otherwise, they're not reliable, they could be anything at any time, they have no integrity.

Leaders especially must exhibit this integrity. They must be reliable and stable. Their team relies upon this. They set the example that the team will certainly follow. A stable, reliable team leader, one who shows consistency and reliability, is necessary for any project's success. Lacking this quality, a leader is a leader in name only.

And, like a wing, a good leader is flexible. The leader in name only will say, not without reason, that the system works and shouldn't be changed for every accommodation. This is not an uncommon nor an unrealistic perspective.

The Twentieth Century existentialist Michel Foucault broke down society into two models, a system model and a process model. Those who followed the system model had good reason to believe that society functioned best as a collection of systems; the judicial system, any government, the penal system, the Catholic church; these things prevailed because they did not constantly change. They had integrity and were stable and predictable. To this end, the individual was not integral nor important. The system was dominant and the individual served as part of these systems; a student in the educational system, a prisoner of the judicial system. This created a functional society.

Others, according to Foucault, follow the process model. The process model focuses on the individual and eschews the dominance of any system. In this model, the individual creates their own system based on the process of examining systems but not succumbing to them. In this model, systems fail and only a process can create the ideal individual. The society with the most ideal individuals is the superior society in this model.

And this also makes perfect sense. In the modern world (and throughout recorded history, really) systems do fail. The penal system has been privatized, creating mass incarcerations and terrible mistreatment. The system known as the Catholic Church was so rife with corruption selling indulgences that Martin Luther's Reformation was necessary in the 1500's, creating the Protestant tradition, of which there are now many sects, each predicated on its own system formed by process.

In general, a fixed-minded individual will lean toward a system-oriented world view. One doesn't question the system; the system is fixed. A growth-minded person is more apt to be a process-oriented individual and resist system thinking as rigid and prone to corruption and failure.

Are you a system-oriented thinker, or a process-oriented thinker? Are you willing to modify your approach and accept flexibility as part of the process, or are you convinced that the rigidity of the system must be enforced? Are you a flexible leader, or a rigid leader in name only?

Did you assemble a team based on their ability or your own? Give this one some thought. A leader in name only wants and needs to remain the leader. Because they generally have a fixed mindset and believe that they are personified by their achievements, leaders in name only cling to their position. Therefore, they are apt to assemble teams which will not outshine them. Negative self-talk and overthinking will lead them to be suspicious of and competitive with their own team. Growth-minded managers will know that their own self-worth is not tied to any particular results, certainly not the positive results of anyone on their team. If anything, that reflects well on the leader. But the leader in name only will become fearful of losing their place, competitive with their best team members. This, of course, is a form of self-sabotage in a number of ways.

On one hand, it may encourage workers to hold back and not do their best for fear of upstaging their insecure boss. This contributes to the overall failure of the project. And that's a pity, because it's the success of the project which matters, it's the success of the sum total of everyone's best efforts which creates the leader's success.

Also, it sets a terrible example that everyone will surely follow. If the leader is insecure, they're unreliable and lacking integrity. His or her team won't be on board any more than you would get on a plane if you knew the wing would tear off in midflight. The team will be insecure and unreliable, they'll suspect and be competitive with one another. This will destroy the chances of success, for the project, the team, and their leader.

A good leader with integrity will always choose the best team members, regardless of any sense of insecurity. Think of the pilot of a big commercial jet. Are they concerned about the navigator taking their job? They shouldn't be thinking of that even for an instant. His or her only concern must be the safe delivery of their passengers to their destination. That's all. The good surgeon doesn't put together a team of lesser technicians for fear of his or her own career. The best surgeon has the best support because their only concern is the success of the operation, the life of the patient. Anything less and they're a doctor in name only.

Are you a leader in name only? Did you assemble a team certain not to outshine you or did you get the best possible talent to do the best possible job?

Be decisive. If you are the leader, you must lead. That means being flexible, as we've mentioned. It also means having some grounding in systems as well as processes. Things will happen for which you may not be prepared. Complications arise during surgeries. Unexpected weather patterns can make a flight treacherous. Decisions will have to be made and may have to be adjusted given varying factors. A leader must be ready to act in response to changing influences. A leader may not always be certain of what to do, and a lot may be on the line.

This brings us back to the concept of overthinking. An overthinker may circle around a problem so much that they become unable to act. It's known as *analysis paralysis,* and it's a lot more common than you may realize. A person may spend their entire life not writing that novel, not creating that business, not perfecting that invention, because they couldn't stop thinking and couldn't start acting. This causes negative self-talk, the habit of bludgeoning one's self with reprisals and berating self-loathing which in itself creates an unwillingness to try new things, a fixed mindset, and a series of self-fulfilling prophecies which may cripple any personal or professional life.

The results of such a downward spiral, by the way, include stress and anxiety, poor diet and sleep habits which may result in substance abuse, weight gain, and the ensuing physical repercussions. Heart attacks, stroke, premature death, and suicide are often the results.

The fact is that not every decision will be the right one. Success entails risk, and risk entails failure. Your decision may result in failure, this you must know. But to not proceed for fear of failure is to ensure failure, that is failure; failure to act, failure to decide.

And if your decision results in failure, it can likely be corrected. If not, you'll be able to externalize that and not let it define you as a person. You'll know that the failure will result in a lesson well learned, and that will contribute to your later successes, it's even considered a necessary part of that success.

Are you decisive despite uncertainty, like a real leader, or do you suffer analysis paralysis like a leader in name only?

A good leader considers the input of others. Some people are utterly confident, and confidence is a good thing. But a team is just that, a team, and it thrives when every member's point of view is considered. There could be wisdom from the perspective of a lesser team member, or one higher up on the hierarchy. This goes back to a level of security on the part of the team leader. A confident team leader will welcome contributions from the team without worrying about being outshone by a member of the team. A true leader will value the end result more than his or her appearance as the source of all good ideas. A leader in name believes only he or she knows the correct course of action.

True leaders set the bar high and reach for it. They know this is the way to improve individual and team efficiency, the way to increase the team's abilities. A leader in name only sets the bar low, knowing it will be an easy success. But easy successes are not successes at all, they are the status quo. Success entails risk, and low-bar achievements require little or no risk. That's why they're not really successes, and why they are commonly set by leaders in name only.

Leaders are gentle in their leadership, not overly authoritarian. Some leaders believe a strong hand is important to keep the team members in line. But that kind of leadership only engenders bitterness, insecurity, paranoia, competitiveness, in-fighting, and that makes for an inefficient team and prevents team successes.

THE CHARACTERISTICS OF A TRUE LEADER

We've taken a look at what makes a leader in name only, and by contrast what makes a strong leader. But there's more to being a strong leader than merely not being a poor leader. The true leader has characteristics he or she brings to the job. It's not just a matter of managing, but of strengths of character which allow a true leader to manage wisely and well.

From George Washington to Richard Branson, good leaders are persistent. They accept failure as part of the process of success. They're growth-minded individuals who can separate their own value from the value of their decisions and actions. They know that no outcome is predetermined, and when they do fail, they don't linger on it. They don't let negative self-talk prevent them from trying again, to keep striving toward ultimate success. Harry Potter author J.K. Rowling, Stephen King, Walt Disney, even the Beatles all faced rejection early in their careers, but persistence led them all to be true leaders (Ringo, maybe not so much).

True leaders have insight, especially into themselves. People who achieve are often self-made, and that takes a lot of confidence. But confidence does not mean being deluded into thinking one is a genius at everything and at every turn. Nobody's perfect, and a true leader knows this about themselves first and foremost. In the same way a true leader listens to the members of his or her team, who are the best he or she can find, a strong leader knows that he or she has some strengths and some weaknesses, just like everybody else.

And a true leader takes this into account when putting the team together. A true leader, secure in his or her position and concerned primarily with the success of the project, will hire people who have the skills the leader knows is lacking in themselves. The leader may be a good motivator, but he or she may lack organizational skills or accounting or artistic skills. That's what the team is for, to provide those things. So, the true leader creates a team with skills that are unique to the team, not the leader.

Along these lines, a true leader is an active listener. They digest what they're hearing, they don't just nod and smile. They want new information and they process it, turning it into positive action if possible. The true leader is never condescending to their team either, because they know the information could further the success of the project, and that is what's most important to a true leader. A leader in name only will appear to listen, all the while thinking about themselves or perhaps looking into a mirror, waiting for his or her time to speak without digesting anything which is being said.

Honesty is a crucial trait to any true leader. We spoke of integrity, reliability, but honesty is key to these things. A person whose word of honor is reliable is a person who is reliable. Nobody has integrity without honesty, because they will react in any way which is best for them. Their words and actions come to nothing more but expressions of desire and convenience. Team members will follow the leader's example and be dishonest themselves, with each other and with the team leader. This will almost surely have disastrous results for the project and, thus, for the team. A person who is lacking in honesty has no place on your team or any team, but certainly not leading a team.

A true leader communicates openly and clearly. He or she says what they think without being frank, crass or rude. They know how to say something positive before saying anything negative. They explain their opinions to better educate the team member and so to elicit even better suggestions to come. A leader in name only relies on old-hat empty phrases (*"We're going in a different direction"* or *"I'll know it when I see it"*) or otherwise muddled or confusing instructions or opinions. It may be inspired by a desire to be kind or gentle, but lacking directness is where things go wrong in almost every professional instance. They also reprimand without being degrading or humiliating their team.

A good leader is forward thinking. They don't just rely on old ways of doing things, no matter how reliable or time-tested they maybe. A good leader is up on the latest technologies. Imagine a team manager who doesn't have a mobile phone or can't use PowerPoint or can't open or send email. From Kubla Khan to General George Patton, great leaders have relied upon the newest technologies and the most creative ideas.

A good leader is likewise fixed on the future, of the project and of the team. He or she knows the ramifications of failure or success, of quality work or work that lacks quality. So, a true leader is always looking ahead. Likewise, a good leader does not linger on failure. They learn the lessons from that failure and then they move on, as quickly as possible.

True leaders not only surround themselves with the best and brightest without concern for feelings of insecurity or competitiveness, they guide and develop others, either in their team or not. True leaders know that the strongest team will prevail, that the team can always be made a bit stronger by improving the performance of the individuals in that team. The true leader develops the skills of the individuals on the team, knowing it will make the team's performance better. True leaders also mentor others who are not on their team. This creates professional bonds which can serve the leader well throughout their careers, and serve as good connections for later projects. Mentoring also increases the general quality of work, and while some may see this as helping the competition, others know that when the water level rises, it lifts all boats with it.

True leaders are self-actualized. They have earned their place by fulfilling their own needs, basic, more complex, aesthetic, and even transcendent needs. They have answered the existential questions of their own lives, they know who they are and they have established a strong set of beliefs. These beliefs must include the higher principles of honesty, integrity, humanity, or the leader is a leader in name only. The true leaders share these standards with others and will not tolerate less from members of the team.

A true leader will lead by example. Behavior is always the benchmark of beliefs, and the leader knows that his or her actions are under special scrutiny; from the team, who look to the leader for an example, and to the client, who looks to the leader for results. So, a true leader always behaves in a way which will be a good example and will make a good impression. And, of course, the true leader guides their team to be and do likewise.

A true leader will work alongside the team. True, the manager often has different duties than the members, who have individual creative and administrative duties. The true leader lets them get their tasks done and goes about coordinating and planning. But the true leader is also there with the team, present to answer questions, ready to react to unexpected challenges which may arise. A leader in name only merely appears from time to time to lord over the crew, throw their weight around, then disappear. They see the team as a resource for them, but they overlook the fact the leader is a crucial resource for the team.

Along these lines, a true leader will not micromanage or control their team. Rather, a true leader will inspire their team, encourage, and guide them. The true leader has assembled the best team possible, and they allow that team to flourish. The leader in name only believes only he or she knows best and feels they have to have a hand in every stage, every task. But that leader does not know their own weaknesses or their team members' strengths.

Along these lines, true leaders delegate to the members of their team. They're confident that they've assembled the best team, and they rely on the members of that team.

But true leaders are not afraid to push their team to reach the highest standard. The true leader knows what must be done and is willing to make sure their team gets it done. While not demanding or authoritative, the true leader still has authority and must make demands, not requests. Of course, the true leader balances authority with humanity and knows that demands are made on everyone in the team, the leader included. Everybody must carry their weight, it's the true leader's job to make sure that they do and coordinate those best efforts. After all, if one member isn't doing their best, the overall success of the project is threatened.

A true leader knows how to properly manage time. This will include time off for self-care, of course. It also means watching timelines, requesting time logs from team members if necessary. Because a true leader is responsible for his or her own time, but also the time management of their team members. A true leader knows that time is the most valuable thing in life, as no amount of money can purchase even a tiny fraction of it (save for a medical context, perhaps). Time is the only thing we cannot afford to waste. And, as the old business adage goes, time is money.

A leader in name only is lazy with time, allowing deadlines to go missed or rushing at the last minute to get things done. A leader in name only will allow his or her team to be slovenly with their own time management, to the detriment of their projects' success.

A true leader will hold his team and his- or herself accountable and responsible. Too many people are too ready to blame somebody else for their mistakes. Often others may err, and teammates will judge them harshly, blamefully. But a true leader sets a better example, one which includes taking personal responsibility. A true leader knows that he or she is ultimately responsible for every member of the team, and they set this high example for their team members to follow. The leader in name only will always blame the team for a lack of success and excuse themselves.

A true leader will keep things in perspective. They make measured decisions, neither suffering from analysis paralysis nor rushing into foolish moves. They consider alternatives, they digest the viewpoints of their team or colleagues, and they make their best choices, then take responsibility for them. They're forward thinking, so they know that their choices will have far-reaching ramifications. The leader in name only is impulsive, making uninformed decisions based on their own needs and not on the needs of the project.

BORN LEADERS VERSUS SELF-MADE LEADERS

It really comes down to a question of nature versus nurture, an age-old question which has been the center of philosophical thought and the inspiration for stories from *Pygmalion* to *Trading Places*.

Almost nowhere is the question raised more often than in the arena of leadership. Out of a group of children, all raised more or less the same, a natural leader tends to rise to the fore. This encourages the nature-based perspective. But others would say that children are rarely treated the same way even by the same set of parents, and that some parents may generate more leaders than others based on parenting styles.

The fact is that people are born with different innate skills and talents. Everybody born in the United States may be equal under the law (ideally) but they are not born equal. In fact, since everybody is unique in very specific scientific ways, there can be no true equity. Some are bigger and stronger, others are gifted with genetic attractiveness, some are born with deformities or other physical challenges.

And many would say that leaders are gifted with the qualities they'll use later in life. These qualities might evince themselves as boldness or even youthful aggression, a raw manner of taking control. Leaders are generally intelligent, and intelligence is undoubtedly an inherent quality, genetically gifted to some more than others.

Some are gifted with genius, and their names ring through history; Albert Einstein, Mozart, Stephen Hawking. Though it's interesting to note that these are leaders in their field, though they often worked alone. They were not managers, not leaders of teams. So, following that train of logic, one can argue that inherent intelligence may have nothing at all to do with leadership skills.

Likewise, aggression can become anti-social, which is not the quality of a true leader. Children who are reserved can grow to become adults who can calmy manage others. Many would argue it's a matter of life experience which shapes an individual and prepares them for one role or another in society; a manager or a maker (a specialist member of the team, usually creative in some way) a nurture-based perspective. Though the naturally creative requirements of the maker are generally both inherited and also developed through time and experience.

Most behavioral theories hold that leadership is a skillset which can be acquired, it can be taught and learned. There are countless books, classes, and seminars predicated on that concept, and their success is testimony to their effectiveness. If people are learning these skillsets to become better leaders, then leadership can be learned, and leaders made and not born.

A growth-minded leader knows that leadership is, like most things, a process. It can and should be refined and improved with time, results and efficiency made even better. This also speaks to the nurture-based side of the argument. Every military in the world engages in leadership training, it's both how and why they move up through the ranks.

Leadership is really an art, and like all the arts it must be learned. True, some geniuses like Mozart can do it virtually from birth. But we're not Mozart. We may have some innate skill, but in general we have to learn and develop that skill through years of painful development and instruction.

Leadership may also be a matter of timing. One may find one's self in the position by happenstance. The true leader is prepared to lead when the moment arises. The leader in name only will either panic or become swelled with egotistical power and delusions of grandeur.

Think of the great leaders in history: Mahatma Gandhi, Nelson Mandela, Martin Luther King Jr, Abraham Lincoln. These were leaders who didn't seek fame or wealth. They were selfless, loving of people, and of justice. They had high standards, integrity, and the courage of their convictions.

The truth is more likely to be, like most truths, comprised of various circumstances. Like most contests of nature and nurture, the answer is, frankly, a bit of both. Some people are gifted with the necessary gifts of leadership, and those can always be refined, and other aspects of leadership can and must be learned through instruction.

The Pareto principle is also known as the *80/20 rule*. Named for economist Vilfredo Pareto, the 80/20 rule tells us that about 80% of effects happen as a result of roughly 20% of the causes. It's confusing, but to make it easy, the rule suggests that a true leader is 80% made and 20% born. However, studies conducted out of the University of Illinois support research that leadership is 70% learned and only 30% genetic.

Leaders apply skills and knowledge in what is called *process leadership*. But It's also a fact that traits can affect our actions, known as *trait leadership*. Leaders carry out this process by applying their leadership knowledge and skills. It's a combination of both that makes a true leader.

WHAT KIND OF LEADERSHIP STYLE ARE YOU USING?

Whether or not or to what extent a leader is made or born, they usually adopt a certain style. They can even be generalized, as the patterns seem to come down to seven leadership styles.

The first is the autocratic style of leadership. This is the most authoritative style of leadership, a my-way-or-the-highway arrangement. A lot of people with military backgrounds may assume this style of leadership, as strictly following orders is part of their training.

But this kind of leadership style is generally fixed-minded and not open to the contributions of others. If often fails to take into account the leader's strengths or, in this case, their weaknesses. This old-fashioned way of leading isn't as effective in the modern era, though some people do still swear by it. Not *my* boss, luckily.

Those who lead in the bureaucratic style are similar to autocratic leaders. They expect the team to follow the rules the leader has set. But the autocratic leader emphasizes his or her own place at the head of the team. The bureaucratic leader, you may have guessed, emphasizes the team as a whole and relies more on the team. This *laissez-faire* hands-off approach can be efficient, but it can also lead to inefficiency, the hallmark of any bureaucracy.

The authoritative style, sometimes called the *visionary style,* also sets the pace, but this style engages team members more than the autocratic style, exciting them and gearing them toward greater participation and superior results.

This is a style that emphasizes guidance, not merely leadership.

The pacesetting style is so-called because this leader sets the pace. They set the bar high, they drive their teams hard and fast. This energetic style is effective but can also be tiring and stressful for some employees.

The best management style in these turbulent times may be the agile leadership style. This is similar to the pacesetting style, but has eyes on the long haul. The pacesetting style may be good for quick turnarounds and short-term projects, but the agile style, a bit more laidback, is better for the long-term.

The fourth style, the democratic style of leadership, emphasizes group think a bit more, leaning on the opinions of the team members. Some leaders find this approach to diffuse, but others realize that the leader still has the deciding hand in all matters. That's what the leader is for, after all. But this style allows for more creativity, greater contributions, encouraging a team spirit, and often creating superior results. It makes the work mood a lot lighter than the previous styles as well.

The coaching style puts the most emphasis on the team members, giving them added responsibilities, a higher bar, and actively encouraging, and guiding them. It's a bit like the pacesetter style, though this approach puts even more emphasis on the team members and their contributions. This leadership style lends itself particularly well to mentorship, which has a variety of other benefits.

You may never have heard of the affiliative leadership style. This leader is more than just a coach, even more of a mentor. The affiliative style, which works in conjunction with others such as the democratic style, focuses on the needs of the members outside the strict confines of the project. Emotional needs are considered, for example, not just practical needs to get the project done.

Some feel those things should be left out of the office, that things become too messy. And it's true that an emotional state and a rational state cannot co-exist in the same psyche at the same time, rational thought should always be the focus of the workplace. Emotions, some would say, are for the home. And that would be true but for the fact that humans carry their emotions around all the time, and the workplace can be a stressful experience. That stress often expresses itself as emotion.

But this leadership style can smooth out conflicts and create collaborative relationships in any team. It's an ideal style for a stressful situation.

Ultimately, this style is all about encouraging harmony and forming collaborative relationships within teams. It's particularly useful, for example, in smoothing conflicts among team members or reassuring people during times of stress.

The *laissez-faire* style will be familiar to anybody familiar with history or politics. Born of the French phrase for *leave alone*, this style takes a hands-off approach to leadership. This style delegates more than leads, gives team members the utmost control over their work schedule. The idea is to let the team flourish, though the downside is often disorganization and a scattershot result.

A transformational leadership style is comparable to the coaching style, but it puts more emphasis on the project goal and less on the team member's performance. The transformational leader is more interested in the game than the players.

A transactional leadership style uses incentives to inspire the team; bonuses, prizes, using contests to keep the team fired up. It's a potent tool for mentorship too. It's great for getting the job done, but creative types tend to resist it, and that's a big part of any manager's job.

In situational leadership, the emphasis is put on the situation above the leader, the team, or even the project. Situational theory stresses four styles of leadership. There is telling, which is instructional; there is selling, which seeks to convince; participating, which invites team contribution, and delegating, which de-emphasizes leadership contribution. The situation will determine what kind of leadership is required.

Which leadership style will work the best for you? It depends on you, your team, and the situation. If you're thrown into a crisis and you have to turn things around, a democratic approach will get you the best results from your team. If you're a new manager of a team already in full swing, you might try the *laissez-faire* approach and switch to democratic if things go wrong. You may lead with one style at one stage of the project, maybe pacesetting at the offset to get things off right, then easy back into an affiliative approach as the office runs along from project to project.

Again, know your strengths. Are you an easy-going type? Affiliative may be right for you. Are you more of an outgoing personality? Maybe the coaching style would be more effective than the autocratic style.

Just keep in mind that there are different styles, and know which one you're employing and why. Don't just wing it. Be aware, be strategic, learn to read when one leadership style will be more effective than another. During times of crisis, you may choose the affiliative style, but only in those times.

If your leadership skills aren't as effective as you'd hoped in one style, figure out why and make improvements. Hopefully, you're growth minded enough to know that everything and everyone can and will likely be improved with time and experience.

Like all skills, leadership skills should be practiced. Don't fall into the trap of thinking you've nailed it. Skills can atrophy, they have to be kept loose, fresh in your mind's so-called *muscle memory* (a term athletes, dancers, and musicians use for a repeated muscular movement which becomes second-nature).

Whatever leadership style you employ, be genuine. Let it come from some real part of you. Don't pretend to be an authoritarian if that's not you. Don't try to coach someone if it's just not in you. And it should be. We all have various facets of our personality which we don't often employ. Discover yours.

EVOLVING TO A LEADER YOU WISH TO BECOME

As we've seen, true leadership is a skillset reliant upon certain personality traits and strengths of character. There are different leadership styles, each of which has strengths and drawbacks. Knowing what type of leader you wish to become is central to becoming that leader. So too are the tools and techniques you'll be reading and learning about in this book. Now that we know what a leader is and who can become one, let's take a closer look at the building blocks of a great leader.

2

THE BUILDING BLOCKS OF A GREAT LEADER

BECOMING A TRUE LEADER IS A PROCESS

We've already seen how leaders are not born, they're made (well, they are born, but not as natural born leaders). Desire and willpower can make an effective leader of just about anyone, experts agree. It is an ongoing process of education, study, experience, and training.

As we defined it, leadership is the process of influencing others to accomplish some objective by means of coherent and cohesive organization. We find it in all facets of our lives; professional, social, and familial.

We've looked into the qualities of a true leader, and of a leader in name only. True leadership requires influence, not power. It requires others, it's not a solo practice.

A leader needs followers, one of the building blocks of any leader. And the true leader knows that different people need to be led differently. Some require a bit more pampering; others bristle at it. But followers there must be, and they are crucial to any leadership. Without them, there's no leadership at all. So, a true leader must always keep in mind how important their followers or team really are.

Clear, healthy communication is vital to being a good leader. That only makes good sense, as the team is so critical to the leader, and communication so vital to their interaction. Learn to improve your communication skills to be the best leader you can be.

Situations are critical parts of being a leader. Situations happen, no matter where you are or what you're doing, it's a situation. So, this is part and parcel of leading. The effective leader must take the situation into account when leading. A conference room is a different situation than a burning building and should be treated as such. The latter is no time for the affiliative approach to discuss emotion. That's a good approach for after everyone's made it out alive.

MANAGEMENT OR LEADERSHIP?

There's a subtle but important difference between leadership and management. The main function of management is to produce *consistency* and order through deliberate processes, including organizing, budgeting, planning, staffing, problem solving, and more.

The main function of leadership, on the other hand, is to produce *change* through a series of processes, such as aligning people, inspiring, and motivating. One may lead through change, but manage the status quo.

While leadership's main function is to produce movement and constructive or adaptive change through processes, such as establishing direction through visioning, aligning people, motivating, and inspiring.

LEADER OR BOSS?

The boss has power, that's true (it's also known as *assigned leadership*). But this can be a leader in name only. The true leader makes their followers want to accomplish their goals, not merely to feel that they have to comply with the boss' demands (also called *emergent leadership*).

EMERGENT LEADERSHIP VS. ASSIGNED LEADERSHIP

So, to be a good leader, you must be more than just a boss, more than just a manager. You must be respected for your ethics and integrity; you must inspire others with a strong vision of the future.

THE PRINCIPLES OF LEADERSHIP

In 1983, the US Army presented the eleven principles of leadership. Any true leader knows them, incorporates them, and now you can too!

Some of them we've already covered, including know yourself and seek self-improvement; be well-trained and experienced, take responsibility and develop that same sense in members of your team, act in a timely but reasoned manner, lead by example, know your team, communicate clearly.

But you will also want to train as a team if you can. Let a new member be trained by the team as they go. Develop and maintain a team spirit, remind everyone that the end result is what's important, not the contribution of any single member.

The US Army stresses the three concepts of leadership: *Be, know, do.* They know who they are, they know their job and the people around them, they do what they must to achieve the goal. It's a good thing to keep in the back of your head.

A true leader exerts an influence on the environment, and they do this with three distinct actions. They establish; performance standards and goals for their team, values for their company or organization, concepts of people and the business they do.

Standards apply to strategies, plans, productivity, reliability, quality, leadership. Values apply to the concern the business has for its customers, employees, investors, and the environment. Concepts apply to products and services offered and the processes and methods of conducting business.

The combination of these three things define how a company is seen, by customers and competition alike. It defines roles and relationships, rewards, and rites within the company.

Roles are, basically, positions within the company which have defined expectations of behavior and productivity. Every team has roles; one the writer, another a graphic artist, the other an engineer, yet another an accountant. Every role has its place, every member of the team has a function.

Relationships depend on the task given to a certain role. Some are isolated, some require more interaction. But no matter how isolated a worker may be, they still must be led effectively.

CULTURE AND CLIMATE

Roles and especially relationships on a team or in a company are affected by both culture and climate. Every company has its own culture. Some are more modern, with offices filled with toys and ping pong tables and other things to create a fresh, young, creative feel. Others are more traditional. This will have an effect on relationships between roles.

Think of the climate as the general feeling which arises from the culture. A newer approach may create a fresher, more easy-going climate, but that may not be best for productivity (though it may do wonders for your ping pong game). Traditional cultures in business may produce a stuffier climate, not conducive to creativity.

Know the climate and culture of your situation and you'll be better suited to lead it correctly and effectively.

Climate and culture can both apply to ethical standards, environmental considerations, even stock payouts. But climate may change and culture is a more enduring concept. The climate may change with an economic downturn, though the cultural model of the company will endure.

Leaders are unlikely to be able to sway the culture of the company, which is generally determined by the company's founders. Unless the leader is the founder, there's somebody else's vision to serve here. But managers and true leaders do affect the climate of the office, and that is one of the true leader's primary functions. Put your focus there when managing or leading.

Other researchers have found more building blocks of great leaders. They often challenge the systems they work with. They're process-oriented thinkers. They inspire the idea of a shared vision, and they inspire others to act accordingly.

5 THINGS EVERY NEW & EXPERIENCED LEADER CAN DO TO BUILD ESSENTIAL LEADERSHIP HABITS

Making the most of your possibilities as a leader means making the most of your own skills. A true leader knows that leadership is an ongoing process. As we've discussed, they include active listening, emotional intelligence, a growth mindset, conducting purposeful conversations, asking questions, being a good coach.

Bad habits which prohibit true leadership include unrealistic expectations. Don't expect supersonic results overnight. Don't expect Herculean results from mere mortals. The best results are often neither quick nor linear, there's not a straight path to success. Often enough, it's a twisting path.

Successful leaders focus on who they want to become, not what they want to achieve. I know this is counterintuitive, and I've been asserting the virtues of putting the results of the effort above the qualities of the individual.

But one does not set out to complete one project, save one patient, or to file one tax return. One sets out to do this continuously, and that has to be kept in mind. It's still imperative to keep a project's success in mind, but it's a matter of perspective. Overall success is achieved through a series of smaller successes. If you're going to be a leader, you're best served to set out on a deliberate course to become a leader.

One building block to great leadership is the understanding between the difference between action and motion. That may be something you've never considered, so let's take a closer look. There's much to be revealed.

Understand the difference between action and motion. Motion is a feeling we get from taking action. But motion does not entail the risk of failure, action does. Still, motion requires action. The trick is to know the difference.

Your risks occur when you take action, your rewards occur when you experience motion.

One habit all leaders seem to develop is reading. It excites the mind; it keeps a person forward-thinking. It's an invaluable resource of information which no YouTube video can replace. And with Kindle, reading is faster and cheaper than ever. Gone are the days of musty bookshelves or cardboard boxes full of books. Almost every book ever written is at your fingertips, in just about every language still used on Earth. And with over half the book market devoted to non-fiction, much of which is self-help, there is a plethora of data to absorb, almost all of which will be new to you and a lot of it applicable to your situations in life.

Leadership also means being generous with praise. Morale is crucial to teamwork, and true leaders know this. Not only should a leader not be competitive or insecure about his or her team, the true leader builds up their team and acknowledges their efforts.

Positivity is a key building block of any leadership. All of the leadership styles are predicated on the concept of positivity. Nothing can happen in a climate of negativity.

Rest is one crucial aspect of good leadership which often goes overlooked. It's vital to an individual's mental and physical health, and to the health of any team. A leader must be well-rested, and he should see to it that the members of his or her team are well-rested as well.

True leaders likewise make their physical health a priority. Regular exercise and a good diet have a positive effect on every aspect of a person's life. And a true leader leads by example. Any good leader would want their team to be physically and mentally fit, and so they must also be that, even more so. Also, there's more responsibility on the shoulders of the leader, and so he or she must be physically fit.

One practical things leaders tend to do is plan their next day in advance. They make to-do lists, and know first thing in the morning what they're going to do. It gives them drive, purpose, organization, and it sets a great example for their team, who should all do likewise.

RESPECT

Respect; it can take a lifetime to earn and only seconds to lose. It's the basis of sound leadership. But how does one earn the respect of others? It's easy enough to see that practicing the qualities of a true leader, honesty and integrity, clear communication and selflessness, will earn the respect of others. But there's another way to think about it, the *12 Cs of respect.*

True leaders *care* about the feelings of others. They show *conviction* and they do it with *clarity* and *confidence.*

True leaders show *courage* in the face of risk and uncertainty and *commitment* to their standards and to their clients and also to their team. They're open to *collaboration.* They *communicate* openly and with *candor, courtesy,* and *credibility.*

The most effective managers know that good team members are supported by their own sense of achievement, responsibility, recognition, and advancement. The best leaders also know that they are in a position of power. They know how to wield that power, and where it comes from, or what kind of power it is. We've touched on some different types of power, but let's take a closer look.

THE SIX SOURCES OF POWER

1. Legitimate power, or positional power, is generated from their role in the company. This is a formal authority; branch managers or sports team coaches.

2. Referent power derives from the individual's ability to attract others and to earn their loyalty. Many managers and team members have this power. Referent power often arises from a personal trait, likability, or charm, as these are at the root of interpersonal influence.

3. Expert power draws on a person's knowledge and skills. It's a narrow source of power, but it's particularly potent when their skill sets are especially valuable to the company.

4. Reward power is derived by one's ability to dispense rewards. Common rewards include pay increases, extra time off, or other promotions.

5. Coercive power is the flipside of reward power, given to those who can dispense punishments instead of rewards. Often this power and reward power are imbued in the same individual. Rewards are usually the favored motivator, as this creates a healthier climate in the workplace.

6. Informational power is wielded by those with access to information. The gatekeepers of data in this day and age wield more power than they realize. Information can be used in transactional exchanges of various sorts. Information is power.

We've taken a deeper look at what makes a true leader. Now, in the second section of this book, more skills which are even more highly regarded than IQ (which, honestly, is just about *all* of them).

LEADERSHIP SKILLS TEST

Here is a research-tested test of your leadership skills. Answer on a scale of one through five, where one is the lowest (no) and five is the highest (yes).

- I always try to see another person's point of view or perspective before giving feedback.
- I don't like breaking a big project into smaller portions.
- I don't take the time to evaluate strategies or progress of the past, I'm more interested in my own perspective and solutions.
- I'm an authoritative leader, it's my way or the highway.
- I believe superior performance and hard work should be recognized and rewarded.
- I can't maintain a positive attitude; it feels fake to me.
- People expect me to give them hope when things go wrong, but I'm just not feeling it.
- Long-term goals are important to me, they bring me more happiness than momentary satisfaction.
- I'm a generally positive person, even when the going gets tough.
- I find it hard to deal with stress.

- I'm eager to follow up one success with another, and I'm excited by new projects.
- Disappointments upset me.
- I tend to blame myself when things don't go as I'd hoped.
- A good manager follows their own vision and doesn't need the contributions of others.
- Employees are trustworthy, for the most part.
- The team leader sets the example of behavior for others in the team.
- I often get angry at things other people don't seem so offended by.
- The harder I work, the harder my team members are likely to work.
- I'm confident in my actions and decisions.
- I'm not really sure where my organization is headed. I keep my eyes on the next deadline.
- Managers should lead by example.
- There's no shame in losing.
- I have a positive influence on others, how they perform, and how they approach their performance.
- I know my team pretty well, what each one is good at and what their weaknesses are.
- Even if I know my team, I don't invite their advice. It only causes problems when I don't use them.
- A good leader harnesses the power of the team.
- Ideals are more important to me than profit.
- I can't manage to prioritize things; they all seem equally urgent to me.

- I do not trust anybody.
- People don't seem to follow my lead.
- I try to argue my case, but I'm just not good at swaying others.
- Brainstorming brings out the best in me creatively.
- Sometimes I feel great, then I'm suddenly thrown into a pit of despair.
- When I lead a meeting, everybody leaves psyched and ready to get back to work.
- I'm not easily discouraged.
- I know my company's mission statement and let it guide my decision-making.
- I stay in touch with my company's evolving place in the business world, changes going on at every level.
- I'm comfortable asking for the feedback of others.
- I have no trouble showing my gratitude for positive contributions and good performances of others.
- Details tend to distract me.
- I don't understand the term, *Thinking outside of the box*. What box?

Don't worry about your score. You'll know by your answers where you need to shore things up to improve your leadership skills. Now let's move on to emotional intelligence.

II

EMOTIONAL INTELLIGENCE

3

UNDERSTANDING EMOTIONAL INTELLIGENCE

IS EMOTIONAL INTELLIGENCE REALLY MORE IMPORTANT THAN IQ?

You've heard the term IQ all your life, but you probably don't know that it stands for *intelligence quotient*. It's a measure of your relative intelligence. EQ, on the other hand, stands for *emotional quotient*. It's a measure of your relative emotional security and control, how you manage yours or others imagination.

There's a standardized test to measure a person's IQ, but not one to measure a person's EQ, so they're hard to equate. But they can be compared. An IQ score of 70 or below is considered an intellect with a disability, 145 is near to the genius level, 180 is the top possible score.

But there's no way to measure your EQ.

And research demonstrates those who lead well and perform well have high IQs and also adequate emotional intelligence. Both are necessary to act and react in the fast-paced corporate world of the 21st Century.

Unlike the IQ, the EQ isn't particular merely to the individual. It breaks down into two components; internal and external, how we deal with our own emotions and also how we deal with the emotions of others.

As regards the management of one's own emotions, there are three hallmarks of emotional intelligence. Self-awareness, in which you understand your own moods and emotions and what effect they have on others. Self-regulation is the ability to control those emotions and impulses, to think before you act. Motivation is the third hallmark of self-emotional intelligence. Motivation is a kind of passion which is more internal, based on inherent propensity to achieve, an internal drive, more than external factors like utility, other people, or the influence of your surroundings.

That's all for the internal part of emotional intelligence. What about the external quotient?

Externally, your EQ measures your management of others' emotions and your own emotional expression. We can break our external EQ down. Social awareness, understanding other peoples' emotional makeup and how they react to your emotional expressions. Social regulation, on the other hand, is how you influence the emotions of others.

TalentSmart researchers assessed over 2 million workers and found that just 36% of them could accurately assess their own emotions as they happened.

There are two more components of external emotional intelligence. Empathy, the ability to share the emotions of others, is a crucial part of emotional intelligence in the external. Likewise, basic social skills are necessary. These include communication and listening skills.

One company, selling insurance, found that their sales agents who lacked empathy, self-confidence, and initiative, all evidence of emotional intelligence, averaged less than half the sales of those who demonstrated those qualities.

The lack of emotional intelligence can have devastating effects in the workplace. Stress and anxiety are always lurking in the shadows of any office, and a leader lacking emotional intelligence will miss the signs and may allow those festering challenges to affect productivity and efficiency. Passive/aggressive interaction, jealousies, resentments, and other destructive sentiments are likely to run wild and create a toxic climate in the workplace. It creates disorganization and mayhem and may tear a team apart.

And, unlike the IQ, a person's emotional intelligence can be increased. A leader can adapt emotional intelligence, refine it, by being more self-aware and communicating more clearly. One study found that roughly half of children enrolled in the public-school system's Social and Emotion Learning program (SEL) had higher achievement scores and 40% demonstrated improved grade point averages.

EMOTIONAL INTELLIGENCE IN EVERYDAY LIFE

Emotional intelligence is quite common in everyday life. When a child comes to you with a scraped knee, you use emotional intelligence. If a coworker is scorned or reprimanded by your boss, they require your emotional intelligence. Even watching a soap opera on TV engages one's emotional intelligence.

But it's especially important to keep emotional intelligence in mind in the workplace. There are rarely family bonds there, probably not as many office romances as one would think. That means the connections aren't as strong in the workplace and they can become easily frayed. Competitiveness, insecurity, and other factors make the workplace especially vulnerable to the kind of anxiety and stress that go along with a lack of emotional intelligence. The EQ is especially important in the workplace.

Greater emotional intelligence benefits the leader by increasing internal awareness, empathy, self-regulation, and collaborative communication. Benefits to the company include better team management, reduced stress, improved company climate, more effective planning, and better results.

And it really should go without saying that emotional intelligence is crucial not only to workplace situations, but personal, familial, and romantic; every facet of life requires emotional intelligence.

MORE ON THE FIVE PILLARS OF EMOTIONAL INTELLIGENCE

We've looked at the five pillars of emotional intelligence; self-awareness, self-regulation, motivation, empathy, and basic communication/people skills. But how can these things really improve our lives? We've seen some examples, such as improving the climate and productivity in the workplace. And we know the same emotional intelligence is required in other areas of modern life. So, let's take a closer look at emotional intelligence outside the workplace.

We've mentioned emotional intelligence in the home. Besides the workplace, emotional intelligence is most important in the home. Only the fact that so many daytime hours are spent in the workplace, and that it's a place of frequent action and crisis, make the notion of emotional intelligence so important.

But the home is really no different. Interpersonal conflicts, unexpected crises, matters both urgent (time related) and important (goal related) arise constantly and need to be managed. When children are in the family, this is even more important. Children have less emotional intelligence and it's up to their parents, the team leaders, to manage their emotions well. If not, the damage can be severe and far-reaching. A child who does not learn emotional intelligence may grow to be an adult who lacks it as well. It's up to the parents to raise an emotionally intelligent child, and to do that they must first be emotionally intelligent. A good parent, like any true leader, leads by example.

There's also the very practical matter of running a happy home. A home in which children are fighting with each other, parents are fighting with each other, or parents are fighting with the children is not a happy home. The children will be raised to behave that way as adults and to raise their own children in a like fashion. If this sounds like your family, know that you can break the cycle now by improving your own emotional intelligence and then increasing the emotional intelligence of those around you through guidance and education and, well, emotional intelligence.

Since stress and anxiety have such detrimental effects on one's physical and emotional health, it's important to note the connection between emotional intelligence and physical or emotional wellbeing. Lack of emotional intelligence allows stress and anxiety to flourish, and they have recorded effects on sleep and eating patterns, causing malnutrition and weight gain and depression, which can lead to substance abuse. These are all proven to cause psychological complexes, mortal disease, premature death, and suicide.

So emotional intelligence is crucial to a long and healthy life.

Emotional intelligence also has an existential benefit. The existential questions of identity and purpose are best approached with emotional intelligence. These aren't mathematical equations, after all, but questions about the meaning of life. They plumb the very depths of the mind and soul, and intellectual intelligence is not enough to find a satisfactory resolution.

In fact, the very concept of success itself is predicated on emotional intelligence. Because those who have it enjoy a smoothness, a functionality in life which naturally leads to increased socialization. That leads to opportunities and those are the gateways to success. Emotional intelligence is something others pick up on, especially if they are the sources of the emotional crisis. Emotional intelligence engenders gratitude and respect, and those are the qualities which lead to opportunity and the success which may follow.

ARE YOU EMOTIONALLY INTELLIGENT?

We've already touched on a few of the hallmarks of emotional intelligence; willingness and desire to succeed and to help others succeed, empathy, self-awareness, passion.

But if you are to be truly emotionally intelligent, you also need curiosity. Self-awareness of one's deficits and passion for knowledge and self-improvement create curiosity about new information, better methods. Curiosity is the hallmark of a growth-minded individual, which all true leaders are. True leaders are also emotionally intelligent.

The emotionally intelligent should have an analytical mind too, in order to process the causes of their own emotions and the emotions of others. Remember that emotion is not rational, but reason can undo emotion. Therefore, the true leader and the emotionally intelligent know when to reason, they can analyze cause and effect and better manage their own emotional expressions and how to deal with the emotions of others.

Those with emotional intelligence also have a kind of faith. It's not religious faith necessarily, though that may come into play. It's a matter of having faith in one's own emotional intelligence. Once one is emotionally intelligent, they must utilize that intelligence in a practical fashion, and that takes discipline, mastery, and confidence. The emotionally intelligent have faith that their EQ will serve them and others well, and they have faith in the techniques which are the hallmarks of EQ, and other communication techniques presented in this book. And there's no reason for the true leader not to have faith, as these techniques are research-driven and time-tested.

Needs and wants are imperative to consider when looking at emotional intelligence. Abraham Maslow's hierarchy of needs illustrates which needs are basic (food, drink, shelter) and which are psychological (love and belonging) and some which are related to self-fulfillment (aesthetic or spiritual or other self-actualization needs).

Wants, on the other hand, are indulgences which may bring pleasure but which are not necessary. A bigger house, a fancier car, the latest iPhone are all wants, not needs. The emotionally intelligent know the difference, but the emotionally unintelligent do not and will often confuse the two. They may need a fancier car or the new iPhone, or at least they think they do.

The emotionally intelligent are generally optimistic, because they're confident in their approach and they have a keen understanding of those around them. This leads to a general positivity and is conducive to effective leadership styles such as coaching and democratic styles.

The emotionally intelligent are often adaptable, as they have their core standards well-grounded and they know they can handle any unexpected crisis which may throw their team into emotional disarray. The emotionally intelligent are also agile enough to know when to change course, to admit when something isn't working or when something else could work better. They accept this without regard to their ego or personal insecurities, as any true leader would do. Like everything about emotional intelligence, this is as critical in the home or in social situations as in the workplace.

The emotionally intelligent tend to be shape-shifters, adaptable to different circumstances and situations. Emotions tend to be chaotic and may erupt out of nowhere, and so the emotionally intelligent can quickly adapt to a new situation and accommodate it appropriately.

Emotionally intelligent people are very rarely perfectionists. Generally, growth-minded individuals, those with emotional intelligence realize that perfection is rarely attained, and that to be a perfectionist is to suffer from overthinking and negative self-talk and a fixed mindset which are all antithetical to emotional intelligence.

They're generally grateful. The emotionally intelligent have prioritized what is important (health, strong social ties, self-actualization) and what is not (material wants or ego gratification). So, they're grateful for what they have instead of desirous of what they do not have. This is especially potent in family, social, or workplace situations, but it is also crucial to the individual and their inner peace, though that's not what we're focusing on here.

The emotionally intelligent don't seem to get easily distracted. Once again, it's about priorities. The emotionally intelligent know what's important and they stay focused on that, whether it's the task at hand or the emotional tumult of a coworker or team member.

Emotionally intelligent people generally have well-balanced lives, with fair amounts of work and play, social and private time. This is because they're more confident than most, less insecure, and more capable of achieving their tasks to relieve the need for overwork.

The emotionally intelligent tend to embrace change, they don't fear it. Their confidence allows them to see the opportunity in the perceived crisis. The growth-minded true leader with emotional intelligence knows that change is both necessary and unavoidable and looks forward to the positive results the change may bring.

Do you have these qualities? Are you lacking in some but not in others? The more of these qualities of emotional intelligence you have, the more effective a leader you'll be, and the happier a person too.

MEASURING YOUR EMOTIONAL INTELLIGENCE

As we've said, there's really no standardized test for EQ as there is for IQ. But if we can put a man on the moon, we can measure emotional intelligence. Leave it to some of the cleverest minds in modern psychology to give us just about everything we need to get the job done. So, if you want to know just how emotionally intelligent you are (or aren't) then read on.

There are several institutionalized tests for EQ, but no single standard. The EIQ:M creates a profile of seven emotional competencies. The EI Report is part of the OPQ Expert System. The Bar-On EQ-i is called a *self-report measure* for varying purposes. Others are other-reported (based on Q/A and involving a questioner or tester) or ability measured (tests of skill or knowledge). The MSCEIT measures ability. The EI-360 test is used for career management and development.

We've included some sample questions from some of the leading tests to set you off on a new understanding of yourself, of others, of your world and everyone in it.

Ask yourself and then answer with a simple *yes/no* answer or on a scale of one to five, where one is the least positive (a *no*) and five is the most positive (a *yes*).

- I recognize my own emotions as soon as I experience them.
- I often lose my temper in times of frustration.
- I am told that I am a good listener.
- I can calm myself when I'm feeling upset or anxious.
- I organize groups well.
- My long-term focus is hard to maintain.
- Frustration and unhappiness often inhibit my decision making.
- I know what my strengths and my weaknesses are.
- I try to avoid conflicts and/or negotiations.
- I do not enjoy the work that I do.
- I encourage feedback and digest it reasonably on what I do well.
- I often review my progress on long-term goals.
- I'm often confused by other people's emotions.
- I don't build rapport well and find it hard to bond with others.

- I consider myself an active listener.

Now try these samples from yet another EQ test, using the same answer style. Consistency is key.

- I know when not to talk about my personal problems with others.
- When facing obstacles, I reflect on previous similar experiences and take comfort and renewed passion from them.
- I don't expect to fail, not even on the first try.
- People don't often confide in me.
- I find it easy to understand non-verbal communication, such as body language.
- I'm in control of my own non-verbal communication.
- Major life events have given me pause to reflect and reconsider my priorities.
- My mood effects my perspective.
- I enjoy the emotions I feel as they are generally positive.
- I live in the expectation of good things, not bad things.
- I tend to share my emotions.
- I savor positive emotions and can make them last.
- Others enjoy the events I arrange or organize.
- I'm eager for new activities and seek them out.
- I generally make a good impression.
- I can read people's emotions by looking at their faces.
- I can read people's emotions by the tone of their voice.
- My emotions change, but I'm aware of how, when, and why.

- Being in a good mood sparks my creativity.
- I visualize the results of a possible success.
- I freely compliment others.
- Being emotional tends to inspire me.
- I often retreat from a challenge, knowing I'm certain to fail.
- I enjoy lifting people's spirits.

Here are some from the Profile of Emotional Competence (PEC), other good examples of questions you'll find in almost any good EQ test. Answer these honestly for a clearer picture of your emotional intelligence.

- I can't track my rising emotions.
- I don't understand why I often respond so emotionally.
- I know how to influence people's emotions if I need to.
- I know how to convince people's intellects if I need to.
- I know the difference between satisfaction, happiness, and relaxation.
- I am comfortable describing what I think and feel.
- I can calm myself down after an emotional eruption or trying experience.
- I have little difficulty cheering myself up.
- I find it easy to handle my own emotions.
- Others often take offense to the manner in which I express emotions.
- I'm often sad and I don't know why.

There are right answers and wrong answers, but no winning score. That will be for you to decide. If you're deficient in your emotional intelligence, you'll know it by your answers and you'll know where to work harder. Are you lacking empathy or self-awareness? Are you deficient in motivation? Take a look at your answers to these questions and they'll tell you.

Now that you've got a grip on your emotional intelligence, let's look at different ways you can increase that EQ!

4

THE 20 MUST-KNOW STRATEGIES THAT CAN BOOST YOUR EQ

W e know that emotional intelligence, like leadership skills, can be attained and modified and improved. But … how? Here are some concrete, proven methods you can apply in order to increase your own emotional intelligence. You can do them at no cost, with no professional assistance, and the results can be immediate.

We've already talked about understanding your emotions, but now it's time to name them. It's not enough just to have a temper tantrum and then feel badly about it. In order to be in control of your emotions (necessary for emotional intelligence) you must know what emotions you're feeling in order to be able to deal with them properly. Is jealousy the root of an emotional outburst, or frustrated expectations resulting in disappointment? If it's jealousy, ask yourself what you're jealous of, how that makes you see yourself. Ask yourself what productive qualities, if any, do your emotions have. Some emotions can inspire, others detract. Name these emotions, understand what they are and what inspires them. Then you can learn to manage them properly.

Seeking feedback is crucial. It's a fact that we just don't see ourselves the way others do, we're far too subjective about the subject of our own bodies, skill, talents. Oftentimes we have no sense of our own limitations, but just as often we have no sense of our qualities. We're generally harder on ourselves than on others, a condition which causes overthinking and negative self-talk in a fixed mindset. That's why it's so important to ask others for their more-objective opinions. Ask them to be honest and don't take offense. You're trying to improve yourself and we could all use some improving in one aspect of our lives or another. Feedback could well be the key to unlocking your true emotional intelligence.

Reading remains the best way to increase your emotional intelligence. Of course, self-help books like these are invaluable (check out our complete line!) and Kindle makes reading easier and more affordable than ever. But don't stop at self-help books (check out our complete line!) because novels and poetry are great ways to increase your emotional intelligence. Works which are heavy on romance and pondering the existential truths excite the brain to these emotional aspects of life, making any person more sensitive to such things. Go and read anything by the great Romantic poet John Keats, who pondered love and mortality in the three years during which he was dying of tuberculosis and see if you're not suddenly more emotionally aware.

Pay attention to how you behave. Do you get more emotional and less disciplined when you drink? Be aware of this and change your behavior. If you know one person to be a trigger for your emotional mood swings, and you know that certain alcohols (or any) tend to aggravate our behavior, change your situation. Stay out of the room, forego the liquor, or simply exert some self-control.

Take a moment to question your own opinions. This is the exercise of the growth-minded individual. It's possible that opinions have evolved, or that they were never well-founded to begin with. Opinions are too often the result of emotion and not reason. It could be that the reasons or circumstances surrounding the reasons have changed. Review your opinions to root out their cause. Also, questioning your own opinions proves that you are secure in your identity and your ethics, you know they will withstand any scrutiny and will only be strengthened by open-minded reconsideration.

Set time aside to enjoy the positive aspects of life. It's great to be learning from the past and working toward a better future, but all too often we neglect the present. Positive results from team members shouldn't be overlooked, nor should a warm, sunny day. The emotionally intelligent are sensitive to positive energy and they know the value of celebrating it. So, make sure you're not overlooking the positive elements of your project, your team, your family, your friends, and your life.

At the same time, you don't want to ignore the negative. If corrections have to be made, they can be done with kindness and consideration and will be all the more effective for that effort. But to ignore poor results or bad behavior is to guarantee that they will continue, and that's not true leadership, that's being a leader in name only.

Deliberately take time to relax. You may meditate, which many do as a relaxation technique. You may enjoy a hot cup of coffee or tea at some point in the day, but make sure to do it. It prevents burnout and gives you time to reflect, reconsider, to gather your physical and intellectual energies for the tasks to come. Make it ten minutes, whenever you generally find yourself most stressed. In the workplace, this is often late in the morning after a rush of necessary business, or late in the afternoon as the end of the business day looms. For families, watch for these pitched moments in the early morning before school and the hours during or after dinner. These are the times when a relaxation break may be the most valuable.

Along these lines, stand up and stretch at least once a day. Lean back, raise your arms, stretch your muscles for about ten seconds. This physical action of pro-active relaxation has notable effects on the brain. Try it for yourself.

While you're trying new things, try to see yourself objectively. It won't be easy, as we've discussed. Body dysmorphia disorder and reverse body dysmorphia are only two ways that we tend to distort our visions of ourselves. Narcissism, delusions of grandeur, the God complex, anorexia, bulimia, and a host of other harmful conditions and disorders are associated with our inability to be objective about ourselves.

Nevertheless, you have to try to see yourself as others do. You have faults, know them. Others do. You have qualities of character, and you should know these too. And it's not only what, but how much. You may have some talent at one thing, more talent at another, but still not as much at either as somebody else. Know your limitations. Know your habits and inclinations. Know what situations and what people and things trigger what emotions and use that knowledge to manipulate yourself or your circumstance, as we've just discussed.

Keeping a diary is a great concrete step you can take to increase your emotional intelligence. It helps you become more objective about yourself, because it externalizes your thoughts and emotions from your actual, physical self. It's also a way to express yourself to yourself, which is key to emotional intelligence.

Get into the practice of looking ahead to how you will feel later, in the near future. Use the popular if/then technique to ask yourself something like, *"If I drink when this person is around, then how am I going to feel? If I feel badly, then how am I going to behave?"* If you're honest with yourself, you'll know how to modify your behavior in order to better manage your emotions.

Get in the habit of paying attention to your intuition. A lot of people ignore this, to their detriment. Overthinking tends to drown out the voice of intuition. But intuition is born of instinct, and that can often be more reliable and accurate than an over-rationalized position of analysis paralysis.

If you don't already have a weekly or daily schedule, create one. Organization is central to emotional intelligence and everything that goes along with being a true leader. But before you can manage a team, you have to be able to manage yourself. You'll also want to encourage your team members (or family members) to maintain a strict schedule too, but that requires that you lead by example.

Maintain (or begin) a healthy lifestyle. Substance abuse and malnutrition has all manner of ill-effects on brain function, and that's at the heart of emotional intelligence. Lack of sleep is also antithetical to emotional intelligence and true leadership.

Engender trust. If you win trust doing one thing (repaying a debt, let's say) that trust will likely carry into other aspects of that relationship. When the people around you know they can trust you to be emotionally intelligent, they will surely open up more often and more thoroughly, creating a healthier climate. Without trust, no organization can truly flourish. The stress, anxiety, duplicity, and chicanery a lack of trust engenders can be crippling for any project, team, company, or family.

Exercise self-discipline. You're not subject to your emotions, they are subject to you. Don't give into them and burst into a tantrum. Find something else to do, if you must. Feel compelled to explode? Go to the bedroom and punch your pillow, that's a time-tested trick that a lot of people find convenient and effective.

Set some personal goals. This is a great way to keep your mind alert and functioning on a high level. It's a series of challenges which will result in satisfaction and accomplishment. It almost doesn't matter what those goals are; clean the closet, repaint the bedroom, quit smoking, fix the fence in the backyard, resolve your back tax problem. Whatever it is, just do it. Be pro-active and goal-oriented.

Volunteer in some way. It's like on-the-job-training for emotional intelligence, including so many of the pillars (especially empathy). It's a good way to spend extra time, it will broaden your social circle, it offers personal satisfaction, self-discipline, and self-awareness.

Make sure you're approachable. A true leader with emotional intelligence knows that open, clear communication is key to a successful project, team, or organization. And hopefully he or she has adopted a leadership style which leads them to interact with the team. But you don't want to be intimidating around your team, and you don't want them to feel intimidated. You want them to feel that they can approach you with questions or concerns. Do this by being gentle without being weak, demonstrate concern for others, just about everything we've covered in this book so far. But apply them deliberately, in a measured fashion. Mastering the application of these principles is key to being a true leader with heightened emotional intelligence.

We've talked about perspective, but it bears repeating here. Emotional intelligence requires you to be able to see the world from somebody else's perspective. Without that, you have emotional ignorance.

Don't be afraid to share your own experiences. If somebody opens up to you with an emotional crisis, consider sharing one of your own. It lets the other person know that you understand their perspective and share it, that you're empathetic, that you'll do whatever you can for them as you would for yourself.

Another concrete step you can take to increase your emotional intelligence is to immerse yourself in a new culture. Travel, see how other people live. You may be surprised at how much suffering there is in the world, so much to inspire gratitude, empathy. It's a great way to refresh your perspective, to learn to see life through somebody else's eyes. If you can't travel, consider picking a culture and making a project out of it. Read some books, both fiction and nonfiction, watch some videos, think about learning at least some of the language. There's great wisdom in most of the world's cultural traditions, and as a growth-minded person you know the value of learning and growing in your journey of self-actualization.

Another good exercise is to find somebody and indulge your curiosity about them. Call and old friend and ask them about their life, what they've been doing and thinking and feeling. Don't talk about yourself until they insist. This is an exercise in putting the focus on somebody else. And it's a great way to keep your friendship alive (which needs to be done proactively).

One invaluable exercise in building or refining emotional intelligence is to cut off from social media for a while. Sadly, this ever-more-pervasive medium has only stunted our emotional intelligence due to isolation and lack of personal interaction. So, don't just message your old friend on Facebook, get together for lunch if you can. There's no substitute for personal interaction where emotional intelligence is concerned.

You may want to get out into new situations a bit more. A bar, a festival of some kind, anything that will put you into contact with new people. Then demonstrate curiosity about them. You can see how these techniques work together for even greater effect.

WHAT NOT TO DO

Don't get dramatic. Emotional intelligence engenders patience, consideration, reason, not an emotional outburst. Be rational, not dramatic.

Don't complain. It puts you in a position of being a victim, not a leader. Instead, focus on a solution to the problem.

Don't be negative. True leaders and the emotionally intelligent are positive in their perspective and their behavior.

Don't dwell on the past. The past cannot be changed and the future cannot be known. Overthinking is the destructive habit of focusing on the past (what could have been said or done) or the future (what may or may not happen) to the detriment of the present (what might be happening now). So, let go of old hurts, grudges, feelings of resentment or betrayal. Those emotions are toxic and may lead to all manner of psychological and physical maladies.

Don't give into peer pressure. It sounds strange to take that out of a high-school context, but it is a problem which lingers in adulthood for a lot of people. But true leaders and those with emotional intelligence know who they are and what their ethical standards are, and those are the influences which prevail, not trends or fads.

Be aware of your vocabulary. Words have meaning. Make sure you're using the accurate words, forgoing hyperbole. Do not use expletives or racial slurs. Carry yourself with dignity at all times, be reliable in this and demonstrate integrity. And it's more than what you say but how you say it. Enunciate, don't slur your words. Don't sneer to lend subtext to certain words. Your intent will always be clear, so you should be clear about it first. The way you speak speaks volumes.

Respond, don't react. A response is generally intellectual, based on reason and consideration. A reaction is generally a more emotional behavior, and should be avoided. If nothing else, one should act with deliberation and not react without it. But often enough, action isn't necessary, simply a measured, rational response. But do respond, it's part of clear, effective communication and it's the leader's responsibility to communicate with his or her clients and/or team.

So not only can emotional intelligence be increased, but these are some sure-fire ways to do it. But what about empathy? You can refine what you think and how you behave, but can you control what you feel? Let's find out!

5

GOING BEYOND SYMPATHY

WHEN SYMPATHY IS NOT ENOUGH

S ympathy or Empathy?

Both end with the suffix -*pathy,* which translates from the ancient Greek as *feelings* or *emotion. Suffering* and *Calamity* are also associated with the translation.

Sympathy translates roughly as *with feeling.* It's best used to describe a way in which we share another's feelings. We can relate to those feelings, be they good or bad.

But when we actually feel those feelings, we're experiencing empathy, meaning roughly *passion from emotion or feelings."* An empathetic person can feel the emotions not only of a person nearby, but a long-dead artist or playwright or the feelings of a subject in a painting or photograph.

Of the two, empathy is the key to emotional intelligence. Sympathy falls short because it is a rational response, not an emotional reaction. Now that we've got the definition of empathy (and sympathy) straight, let's take a more in-depth look at the concept of empathy. There's a lot more to it than you may have realized!

ELEMENTS OF EMPATHY

First, let's review the elements of empathy, many of which we've already touched upon as empathy relates to emotional intelligence and true leadership.

Understanding others is key, knowing their emotional and reasonable positions, knowing their strengths and their weaknesses, knowing their personality types and how to know which management style will be most effective in managing that type.

Developing others is a hallmark of empathy, the desire to reassure and reconstruct, to help others as much as to help one's self. This includes guidance, mentoring, offering incentives, and rewards for accomplishment.

Having a service orientation is critical. Always keep in mind that any leader's efforts are in some greater cause, and in the modern world that is basically oriented to proficient service. A manager is answerable to their supervisors. The leader's team is answerable to the leader. Everybody's efforts are in the service of the project, of the client. This approach is like going the extra mile and is likely to engender professional respect and fondness.

Empathy leverages diversity. Remember that. Leveraging is about being agile in your interactions. Without violating your integrity, you will be leveraging your behavior a bit with your own supervisor compared to the way you'll behave with your team. The manager is the authority figure in one circumstance, but not in the other. And the true leader and the emotionally intelligent person knows that different situations require different, calibrated responses just as different people require and react better to different leadership styles. So, diversity is an opportunity to the emotionally intelligent true leader.

Political awareness is also key to empathy. If you can feel for the person on the other side of the aisle, especially in this day and age, then you truly are practicing empathy. Hats off!

TYPES OF EMPATHY

Beyond the elements of empathy, psychologists identify distinct types of empathy.

In cognitive empathy, you may understand someone's emotions and thoughts, but that understanding is more rational than emotional. It very much resembles simple sympathy. Emotional empathy is what we think of as empathy in general, though it's also known as *emotional contagion*. It's related to actually feeling the same feelings as the subject, as if the feeling were contagious.

Either cognitive or emotional empathy may lead to compassionate empathy, which goes beyond understanding or sharing and moves onto action to help or reverse the person's suffering.

Affective empathy entails understanding another's emotions and respond appropriately. This is the cornerstone of emotional intelligence.

Somatic empathy goes even deeper, involving a physical reaction. When one person is embarrassed and another blushes, that's somatic empathy.

Let's try another quiz. Answer *yes* or *no* or on a scale from one to five, one being closest to *no* and five being closest to *yes*. Let's find out how empathetic you are. Some may seem familiar, and that's not a coincidence.

- People often tell me their problems, they trust me.
- I'm pretty good at picking up on how people feel.
- I often consider how others feel.
- People tend to come to me for advice.
- I sometimes feel overwhelmed by events in the news or by social situations.
- I try to help those who might be suffering.
- I am good at reading people's honesty.
- I really care about others.
- I find it hard to set boundaries in my relationships.

The ability to empathize seems to be another case of nature versus nurture. And, as we've seen, the true analysis is that both factors contribute. Some people are more prone to emotion, some to reason. For both, life experience takes its toll and creates the sum total, a person either prone to empathy or those not prone to it.

At the most basic level, there appear to be two main factors that contribute to the ability to experience empathy: genetics and socialization. Essentially, it boils down to the age-old relative contributions of nature and nurture. Parenting has as big an influence as genetics where empathy is concerned.

BARRIERS TO EMPATHY

There are things which prevent the proper development of empathy, however. While it can be learned, it may not be and here's why.

Cognitive biases may include blaming others for internal characteristics while considering themselves victims of external factors. This distortion of perspective can be a crucial mistake.

Dehumanization refers to the tendency to let differences of culture lead to a reductive view of a person or culture. The treatment of the Jews in mid-century Europe is an example.

In victim blaming, the victim may be held responsible for the crime, such as the case of a rape victim whom some might claim dressed too seductively for her (or his) own good and was *asking for it.* But nobody buys that.

NEUROSCIENTIFIC AND PROSOCIAL EXPLANATIONS

Though empathy can be learned, much of it does seem physiological and is rooted in the brain. Researchers believe that the anterior insula and the anterior cingulate cortex play a big part in empathetic reactions. There are proven neurobiological components, mirror neurons which mimic emotional responses, to the emotion of empathy.

There's also functional MRI research which indicates that the inferior frontal gyrus (IFG), also a part of the brain, may play a vital role in experiencing empathy. Studies show that brain damage can affect emotional expression.

Sociologist Herbert Spencer suggested that empathy is hardwired into our brains as a way of ensuring social survival, that without it we would be less united and less social, and therefore, less apt to survive. The story of the human race is the story of civilization, after all. Heroism and altruism are also associated with empathy.

DEVELOPING EMPATHY FOR OTHER PEOPLE, EVEN IF YOU DON'T KNOW THEM PERSONALLY

Empathy shouldn't be reserved for friends or pathetic children in late-night commercials to solicit an impulsive donation. In fact, empathy will be beneficial to almost anyone in your life, as empathy affects every strata of your life. Those most affected by your empathy include colleagues and business partners, coworkers and community groups, friends, family, and romantic/intimate relationships.

The famed social psychology researchers Hodges and Myers have described emotional empathy in three parts. They include sharing the felt emotion of the subject as we've described, feeling personal distress in response to that shared pain, and feeling compassion for the person enduring the original pain.

Try attending somebody else's church. That's a good practical way to see a shared experience though somebody else's eyes.

TOO MUCH EMPATHY?

Is it possible to have too much empathy? Surely, one cannot have empathy for everybody all the time, as that would be too draining on any individual's resources. To have one's body endure that kind of constant sensation would rob it of valuable proteins and other physiological resources needed for survival.

Yet the tendency is all too real. Sometimes we care so much that we care too much. This can stifle empathy itself as a matter of simple self-preservation. Those survival instincts are stronger even than our tendency to overthink.

An imbalance of empathy, or a tendency toward sympathy and away from empathy, can be problematic. It's the difference between a leader in name only and a true leader.

DEVELOPING EMPATHY: 5 STAGES AND 5 FACTORS

Stages of empathy development include newborns, infants, toddlers, early childhood, middle childhood to adulthood. Let's take a closer look at both.

1. Newborns are apt to exhibit signs of distress when other

newborns do. One cries, they all cry. It's called reflexive crying or sometimes emotional contagion, which we've already looked at briefly. It's a sign of innate empathy.

2. Infants often have trouble regulating their emotions or managing others' emotions, though they often exhibit great concern for others. Toddlers (14 to 36 months old) begin to evince empathy in behavior such as apologizing. This is also a very emulative phase of growth, where toddlers are experimenting with different modes of behavior based largely on parental or media influences. Fantasy games are common in this stage of development.

3. In early childhood, children experience others' emotional states and also imagine their experiences. This is when, according to *the theory of mind,* children come to understand themselves in the context of other people and society in general. They also get in closer touch with their emotions, thoughts, wants, and desires.

4. From middle childhood and into adulthood, empathy develops significantly (or fails to do so). Perspective taking and empathic concern develop significantly in this last and longest stage of this cycle.

5. Temperament is also a big part of anybody's propensity for empathy. Shy or fearful children appear less likely to engage in empathetic behavior, for example.

6. Parenting is always a major influence on childhood development, but researchers have found a clear link between empathetic parents and empathetic children. This,

like leadership skills and other things covered in this book, is a learned skillset. Most things children learn up to the age of seven years comes from their parents.

6

EMOTION REGULATION IS ONE OF THE MOST IMPORTANT SKILLS YOU CAN DEVELOP

E motional regulation, either automatic or controlled or conscious or unconscious, is the controlled governance of one's own emotions. This includes positive and negative emotions.

Emotional regulation generally involves three separate components: enabling actions which are triggered by emotions, inhibiting actions which are triggered by emotions, and modulating responses which are triggered by emotions.

Emotional regulation is a kind of filter to separate important information. In general, people with higher emotional control or emotional intelligence, have better depression management. Those without significant emotional regulatory skills suffer from mood swings and other detrimental behaviors.

Emotional regulation has been proven to delay a fight-or-flight panic response. It allows time for reason to prevail.

3 KINDS OF FUNCTIONALITY

Emotional regulation is important because without it we lackE functionality. There are three kinds of functionality;

1. Emotional
2. Social
3. Executive

Emotional functionality relates to how you internalize emotion. Social functionality relates to how you express your own emotion and interpret the emotions of others. Executive functionality allows for goal-oriented behavior, including planning and execution.

The first two are easy to understand, but what exactly is executive functionality? Here are some hallmarks of executive functionality:

- Flexibility has come up a lot in this book and for good reason. It's central to functionality of all sorts, true leadership and emotional intelligence too.
- Executive functionality engages the theory of mind, or insight into other people's perspectives.
- Anticipation is the result of recognizing recurring patterns in events.
- Problem-solving is crucial to executive functionality, as is decision making.
- Short-term and long-term memory are pillars of executive functionality.
- Sequencing is the practice of breaking down complex tasks

into smaller manageable units and then prioritizing them in a proper right order. This skill is fundamental to executive functionality.

6 MOST USEFUL EMOTIONAL REGULATION SKILLS FOR ADULTS

As we've seen, self-regulation is the art of pausing between emotion and reaction. We know that emotions react and intellect responds, so the idea is to slow down between emotion and reaction, to insert some intellect into the process to create a response instead of a reaction.

But there's also the notion of *value engagement*. Impulsive reaction may detract us from our core values. In the heat of the moment, we may even act in a way which is contrary to those values. Emotional regulation allows time to reconsider those core values and thereby stick closer to them in our behavior.

The same skillset which allows for emotional regulation was also in play in refining emotional intelligence and also leadership skills. Primary among them is self-regulation. Know what you're feeling and govern from within. Name your emotions and deal with them in the appropriate fashion.

Practicing mindful awareness will not only help you emotionally regulate, but it's a powerful tool in improving your emotional intelligence. Mindful awareness is just what it sounds like, a deliberate sense of wonder about the world, yourself, other people, everything. It's about using that positive, optimistic outlook and gratitude we talked about before and being aware of the positive things around you; a sunny day, a pretty girl, a tasty sandwich. It's a stop-and-smell-the-roses outlook which is sure to help you regulate your emotions, become more emotionally intelligent, and be a better true leader.

When you alter the way you think, that's cognitive reappraisal, and it's a pillar of emotional intelligence and emotional regulation. It's also central to various techniques of mental therapy, including anger management. Situational role reversals and thought replacement are common cognitive reappraisal exercises.

Adaptability is key to emotional regulation. Without emotional regulation, flexibility and adaptability are hampered, changes become crises.

Self-compassion is also crucial to emotional regulation. Often neglected in various facets of life and for various reasons, self-compassion is the parallel of compassion for others. It is a cornerstone of empathy, though most people don't realize it. Some even feel that they should be suffering so others can prosper, it's called the martyr complex. But that complex is antithetical to being an emotionally intelligent true leader.

Some popular exercises in self-compassion include gratitude journaling. Every day, write down the things you're grateful for. It's not complicated, but writing things down gives them power and permanence. It takes them out of the ether and makes them concrete. Writing them and then reading them externalizes them and gives them their own life.

Positive self-affirmations are common to those who deliberately practice self-compassion. They may even address themselves in a mirror. The *Saturday Night Live* character Stewart Smalley (Al Franken) practiced self-affirmations this way to hilarious effect ("I'm smart, I'm worthy, and doggonit, people like me!") but it's a powerful tool for a lot of people.

Breath control and relaxation are also common to those who practice emotional regulation. It gives you time to reason and respond instead of just reacting. Meditation is also popular among those who can regulate their own emotions. Meditating simply means to focus on a certain thing, often one's own breath, to the exclusion of everything else. Some concentrate on a mantra, or repeated word or phrase. Some concentrate on a visual focal point, like a crack in the wall. Some meditate for five minutes a day, some for an hour or more.

Emotional support is a big part of emotional regulation, and that only makes sense. Giving emotional support to others can only strengthen your sense of empathy, and that increased emotional intelligence will allow you to improve your self-empathy as well. This advances emotional intelligence and that contributes to emotional regulation. They all work together.

SCIENTIFIC STRATEGIES FOR EMOTION REGULATION

Cognitive reappraisal is a long-term approach to emotional turmoil. It's not about suppressing the negative emotions, it's about eliminating them. With cognitive reappraisal, one embraces negative emotion in order to understand what created it. Cognitive reappraisal sees the emotion as symptomatic of deeper cognitive processes and focuses on those in order to correct the negative emotional response.

Self-soothing reduces the effects of sadness, anger, and agony brought about by negative experiences. It's the opposite of self-confrontation. It's like using positive self-talk instead of the more common negative self-talk. Meditation is a popular method of self-soothing, and so is masturbation. Most people just go with breathing exercises and maybe reminiscence therapy when at the workplace, however. Others enjoy a massage, a hot bath, indulging in a hobby.

Attentional control is a pillar of emotional regulation. After a reappraisal, attention control is a disciplined way of seeing things from a new perspective. What good is a reappraisal if you lack the discipline to adjust your point of view? If you can't change your perspective, why reevaluate?

Unfortunately, some people just can't manage to do these things and they can't regulate their own emotions. These people are said to suffer from emotional regulation disorder, also known as *emotional dysregulation* (ED). Common symptoms include sudden, unexplained and inappropriate outbursts of anger, passive-aggressive traits or practices, inexplicable chronic pain or illness, self-destructive behavior, inhibited social or professional interaction, and inability to focus.

Poor self-control and hypersensitivity are also common to those who lack emotional regulation. Mood swings in the extreme are common as well, as is depression, stress, anxiety and, irritability.

Psychologists often prefer to manage EDD with dialectical behavior therapy (DBT), often combined with other cognitive strategies. But the prognosis for treatment is generally good. Behavior can be corrected, new behaviors learned to replace the old.

FOSTERING EMOTIONAL REGULATION IN CHILDREN

Emotional regulation is crucial for proper childhood development. But how do we teach our kids to do what a lot of adults cannot? It's actually easier, because children are more pliable and learn more quickly than adults and they lack the imprinted behaviors and perspectives which may inhibit adult growth.

First of all, model the behavior you wish the child to emulate. As in all things and especially in parenting, lead by example. It's the best way to lead and the best way to live. It's also the most effective way to teach.

You may want to deliberately delay response time with children. If they're angry, lead them through a moment of self-sympathy, a moment to create an intellectual response to replace their emotional reaction. You had to deliberately do it for yourself, and you will likely have to be the one to do it for your child, who will likely lack the self-awareness and self-discipline to do it. Do it with them and that will teach them to do it for themselves later in life. It's a gift that keeps on giving.

Focus on the emotional vocabulary of the child. Children are often incapable or articulating their feelings, just as adults are. You went out of your way to name your emotions so as to better understand them.

Do the same with your child, and in so doing you'll teach them to do it for themselves later in life.

You may even make a chart with every emotion along with a facial expression to go along with it. This will help your child visualize and also separate themselves from their emotions. It's also a fun, creative activity that will give you and your child some time together, a shared goal, and the satisfaction of achieving that goal.

Teach your children that actions have consequences. This is key to emotional regulation because the consequences of many actions are emotional responses. An insult may result in hurt feelings, for example. Make sure your children realize that if they punch another kid, that kid may cry and rightfully so. This may create feelings of shame and guilt and will result in punishment.

Make your children aware of things like stress, sadness, anxiety. This will instruct them as to their creation of those feelings in others, and that will help guide them in regulating their own behavior. These are consequences which may derive from your child's actions, after all.

Of course, things with your children may get more complicated than you expect (they often do). Children of different ages react differently to perceived crises. Young children, lacking emotional intelligence, may have meltdowns (so too may adults lacking the same EQ). If these tantrums continue past the age of four, if they become violent, or if they occur often and last longer than 15 minutes, you've got a behavioral problem on your hands. Meltdowns may also be symptomatic of mental illness such as attention deficit/hyperactivity disorder, also known as ADHD.

Meltdowns are caused by so-called *big feelings,* emotions which a child cannot clearly name and identify (much less deal with). But these big feelings can be a problem when a child suppresses their emotions, argues often, makes threats, starts fights, lacks self-control, or has conflicts with authority.

Anger and overexcitement are often associated with mental illnesses and disorders such as ADHD, intermittent explosive disorder, conduct disorder, mood and anxiety disorders, depression, post-traumatic stress disorder (PTSD), and adjustment disorder.

Here are some concrete techniques you may use in dealing with a child who cannot regulate their own emotions:

- To prevent a meltdown, try distracting the child. Move them to a less frustrating situation or activity. Try to meet whatever unexpressed need the child may have. The child can't put a name to it, so it's up to you to know and name their emotions, to know what causes them and to be able to affect it.
- Offer some simple choices to encourage confidence in decision making and lower frustration.
- Actively listen to your child's opinions and concerns. Encourage them to express themselves in this way, as it's key to their own emotional regulation. Validate their feelings too, as they are legitimate whatever those feelings may be.
- Teach your kids what those big feelings are, how to name them and the importance of dealing with them. It's great to

solve your child's frustrating problem on any given day, but you won't always be there to do that for them. What is key is to teach them to do this for themselves, to become emotionally regulated adults.

- But for the moment of crisis, you may want to set aside a safe space where you child can retire for a moment of relaxation and reflection. You do the same thing yourself, hopefully.

- Always communicate clearly with your children, as you would with anyone else. You can't expect them to rise to your expectations if you don't make those expectations clear. A true leader has mastered clear communication and is careful to manage and maintain it.

- Children crave stability, so maintain rituals and routines. Homework after school, brushing teeth before bed, make the bed before school; these are the kind of little exercises in self-discipline that will encourage the bigger tasks of emotional regulation, intelligence, and leadership later on.

- Use schedules and timetables with your kids. It teaches them to do the same and it's a time-tested management tool. All your lives will run more smoothly.

But what do you do during a meltdown, once it's too late to prevent one? The safe place is a good remedy, and there are others. First of all, stay calm. Lead by example here. Speak in a tone which is both gentle and strong, speak from deep in the chest. Declare but do not demand and do not ask. Inquire about the reason for the upset and introduce reason to replace emotion.

After a meltdown, be sure to praise the child for calming down and getting control of themselves; it's a stepping stone to greater emotional regulation, after all. Talk to the child afterward so that you can both digest the details and complexities, the causes and the alternatives. Plumb your child's feelings about the experience, it will help them understand their own feelings and encourages self-sympathy and self-awareness. Talk about problem solving, make a plan to correct things which caused the upset. That's a shared activity with a beneficial goal, a bonding experience for you and your child in which you share positive energy and a positive outcome.

EMOTION REGULATION SKILLS FOR CHILDREN

Here are some time-tested skills any family can work on together:

- First, help your children develop problem-solving skills which use the energy generated by big feelings to create constructive results. These skills fix problems instead of the emotional reaction which only make matters worse.
- Some steps in problem-solving include identifying the problem from the child's point of view, sharing your concerns, working together to make a plan of action, putting that plan into effect, reflecting on the plan's success and modify it for greater future success.
- Teach assertiveness skills, ways a person may declare their needs without being overly aggressive. Teach balanced thinking, to see things realistically and objectively. For kids, books are especially effective ways to teach these skills. There

are mental health professionals who specialize on working with children too. But there are a few more good tips to helping kids with less emotional regulation.

- Make sure they're educated. They can't name their emotions if they don't know the words or what they mean. Teach your children these things, because your local elementary school won't. It's another reason why it's so important that you have a functioning mastery of emotional intelligence; you can't teach what you don't know.

- Resist blameful or shameful language. No person can change how they feel, only how they behave. No emotion should be demonized, merely understood and responded to instead of reacted to.

- As always, be empathetic and an active listener.

- Encourage them toward relaxing activities like exercise and yoga, listening to music, or keeping a journal. Adopt regulating behaviors, such as counting slowly from 10.

DIALECTICAL BEHAVIOR THERAPY (DBT)

Dialectical Behavior Therapy (DBT) focuses on active communication in addressing mental health issues and is particularly useful in treating various personality disorders, such as borderline personality disorder. These are disorders wherein the sufferer may lose control of their emotions.

The idea here is that arousal levels vary with the individual. A child will react differently to a death than a person of middle age, for example. The effects and consequences will vary accordingly. DBT is generally supportive, cognitive (centered on thought over emotion) and mutual (between the client and the therapist).

You may not be a therapist, but you can still do a lot to improve your own emotional management and you can help others do the same. Try the simple techniques you've learned in this book, including identifying emotions, reducing hypersensitivity, and employing stress management.

EMOTIONAL REGULATION EXERCISES & ACTIVITIES

There are several breathing exercises which are perfect for emotional regulation. When you're breath counting, for instance, you're focusing on our breathing, as you would do when you meditate. Breath slowly and deeply.

Slightly different, breath shifting entail putting your hands on your abdomen and over your heart (one each at the same time). You'll be able to feel where your breath is by feeling it. Then shift your breathing downward, from the chest (where it's most likely to be) to your abdomen (where it could and should be).

Breath relaxation is ideal for reducing stress and anxiety and is great for emotional regulation. Not merely focusing on the breath, this practice focuses on the connection of body and mind and visualizes clarity being achieved with every breath. Good stuff.

EMOTIONAL CATHARSIS

We've discussed emotions as being like food; they're necessary for survival, they nourish our lives, but they have to be processed and the residual material ejected or it becomes toxic. One notable thing about EDD is the tendency to hold onto old emotions long past their time. Emotional catharsis allows a client or sufferer to vent suppressed emotions.

But you already have the necessary tools for an emotional catharsis as spelled out in this book. Observe emotions in the raw, unmodified, before you try to change them. Understand them, name them, know them for what they are. Then evaluate your experience and the associated feelings and emotions. Externalize your emotions from yourself. You'll always be yourself, but your emotions will come and go. Name your emotions, seek feedback.

BE MINDFUL OF EMOTIONS

We've already discussed being mindful, or living in the moment with deliberate awareness and gratitude. But there are two types of mindfulness exercises which will definitely help develop proper emotional regulation.

Acknowledgment exercises include observation of behavior and naming thoughts and emotions, as we've discussed. Implementation exercises emphasize non-judgmental thinking and active listening, effective communication and self-expression, and expressions of empathy.

There are also self-awareness techniques which can bring any person greater emotional management. Self-awareness is part and parcel of mindfulness and it's crucial to emotional management.

Every day, ask yourself how you're feeling at any given moment. Be aware of who or what caused it, how you responded. Keep a journal to track your patterns and your progress.

EMOTIONAL REGULATION THERAPY (ERT)

One self-awareness technique is known as *emotion regulation therapy*. This person-centered approach uses mindfulness and parts of DBT, CBT, and other humanitarian approaches to help individuals to identify, acknowledge, and then describe their emotions. It allows for the self-acceptance which results in emotional regulation.

Emotion regulation therapy entail cognitive therapies (thought over emotion) like reappraisal and labeling of emotions. Group therapy may also be effective.

AUTISM AND EMOTIONAL REGULATION

Autism Spectrum Disorders (ASD) is a group of neurodevelopmental conditions which disrupt emotional, social, and executive functionality. Lack of emotional regulation is a hallmark of ASD. Symptoms include communication impairment and impaired social interaction, aggressive or extreme behavior which recurs, low impulse control and poor judgement, involuntary movements and muscular inflexibility or other motor or sensory disturbances.

ASD is often tested with a rating system, listing, visualizing trouble-some social factors which serve as triggers for anti-social behavior.

THE RADICAL ACCEPTANCE WORKSHEET

Psychologists often use the Radical Acceptance Worksheet in DBT interventions. It entails seven subjective questions to gage emotional control and reveal cognitive disruptions. It may prove helpful for you or someone you know! Answer these questions for yourself in the interest of self-awareness.

- Describe a single stressful situation. How did it occur and what affect did it have on you or others?
- Did that situation occur as a result of your behavior? How so? Be specific.
- Did others contribute, either positively or negatively, to the situation? How so? Be specific.
- Did you exhibit self-control as that situation unfolded? Be honest.
- How did you react? Did your behavior impact your emotion?
- Did your reaction have an effect on those around you? How so?
- Would you react the same way to a similar situation again?

THE EMOTION REGULATION WORKSHEET

Now try the questions on the *emotion regulation worksheet.* First, consider a circumstance or situation which was emotionally impactful for you. Now ask yourself:

- What caused the situation?
- What was your interpretation of the event?
- Were your emotions intense? Where would they fall on a scale of one to 100?
- Was your emotion impactful on others? How so?
- Were your emotions impactful on your behavior? How so?
- Was your judgement influenced by your emotions? How so?

We talked about the fight-or-flight response, generally a panic-oriented response to crises. This occurs in the parts of the brain called amygdalae, and there's one of each on each side of the brain. It's an instinctive, primitive part of the brain, where the survival instinct is generated.

The prefrontal cortex, on the other hand, handles logic, reason, along with other high-level functions. Albert Einstein's theory of relativity was generated in this part of the brain, for example.

But the prefrontal cortex doesn't operate as quickly as the amygdalae, and that's where, why, and how emotional reaction trumps intellectual response. Normally, this is fine; we have time to reason things out. But when emergencies or crises arise, there's little time for rational thought and emotional reaction kicks in. It's just the way our brains are wired.

But knowing this means anyone can thwart their natural instincts and deliberately pause to let their brain's cognitive powers kick in. It's the concept of relaxation and reflection we've been discussing, and you can see how it all ties in.

Luckily, you can control your brain as much as it controls you. And there are practical ways to do this!

- Identify problematic behavior
- Identify the emotions which precede that behavior
- Identify emotional triggers
- Become a witness to your own behavior
- Deliberately choose your responses instead of letting instinct dictate them.

THE PROCESS MODEL

The process model is the prevailing emotion regulation theory and it specifies a sequence of emotions include (in this order) a situation, attention, an appraisal, and a response. Every emotion is generated by a situation which commands attention. That attention stimulates an appraisal, and that appraisal initiates a response. For example, a racial remark is a situation which may command your attention, generate the appraisal that such a remark is unsuitable, and that may inspire a corrective response.

You can regulate your emotions at any point in the cycle. You can remove yourself from a situation. You can't unhear what you've heard, but you can divert your attention to something else. But you can change your appraisal by seeing things through another person's perspective and practicing empathy. You can consider your response and choose not to respond at all. Not every stimulus requires or even warrants a response.

True emotional regulation is achieved by accepting emotions as honest as reasonable and externalizing them from the person who has them. Anger is anger, jealousy is jealousy, but every individual who experiences those emotions is unique.

True emotional regulation often requires deliberate techniques and their applications, such as relaxation or other behavior changes. True emotional regulation requires impulse control.

OUTBURSTS ARE HAMPERING YOUR LIFE WITHOUT YOU EVEN KNOWING IT

Sometimes something temporary like lack of sleep or low blood sugar can cause an emotional outburst. More often, however, it's a chronic problem often called emotional liability. It's common to those with brain injury or other pre-existing conditions. They're common to sufferers of borderline personality disorder and other serious mental conditions such as adjustment disorder, oppositional defiant disorder, autism, and ADHD (attention deficit hyperactivity disorder).

The emotional outbursts generally feature fits of laughter or crying, sudden irritability, anger without any real cause, loud outbursts or fits of rage or temper.

Common causes of these emotional outbursts include stress.

What are the causes of being unable to control emotions?

These other disorders and conditions are also associated with emotional outbursts: alcohol abuse, antisocial personality, Asperger's syndrome, bipolar, diabetes, delirium, depression, psychosis, PTSD (post-traumatic stress disorder), schizophrenia.

In general, those who cannot control their emotions exhibit common symptoms. These include fearful of expressing emotions, being overwhelmed by emotion, unexplainable anger, misuse of drugs or alcohol.

The condition can become worthy of medical treatment when the suffer feels that life is no longer worth living, wants to hurt themselves or commits self-harm, hears voices or sees hallucinations, loses consciousness.

PSEUDOBULBAR AFFECT (PBA)

The pseudobulbar affect (PBA) affects people with brain injury or neurological conditions and is known for involuntary bouts of laughter, crying, or anger. It happens as the result of a disconnection between the frontal lobe, which controls emotion, and the cerebellum and brain stem. It can often happen as a result of Parkinson's disease, stroke, brain tumors, multiple sclerosis, and dementia.

Other serious symptoms signaling the need for medical attention include emotions without cause, frequent outbursts, difficulty expressing emotions and constant feelings of anger, sadness, or depression.

Treatments depend on the severity of the condition, but cognitive therapies are often effective. For low blood pressure, try glucose tablets, fruit juice, or candy.

Journal keeping is often helpful. Make an emotional journal and write down when and where you have these outbursts, who is around, what is the cause of the upset. This will help you isolate the causes and control the circumstances and avoid the triggers which help cause the outbursts.

EMOTIONAL INTELLIGENCE TEST

Here's a great applicable test to measure your EQ and show you where you can improve yourself right here and now! Pick one of the two possible answers.

1. My emotions generally have ...

A1: little to no impact on my behavior.

A2: a strong impact on my behavior.

2. I'm usually guided by ...

A1: my values, ethics, and goals.

A2: the values, ethics, and goals of others.

3. Under pressure, I often demonstrate ...

A1: different behaviors than normal.

A2: unchained behaviors.

4. I usually learn most ...

A1: by acting in the present.

A2: by thinking about the past.

5. I usually ...

A1: can laugh at myself.

A2: can't laugh at myself.

6. I usually present myself ...

A1: with power and presence.

A2: with cautious confidence.

7. Facing uncertainty, I'm often ...

A1: decisive and clear-headed.

A2: cautious of making the wrong decision.

8. I express opinions which ...

A1: might be unpopular, but they represent what I think is right.

A2: are popular and widely supported.

9. I generally like to ...

A1: face new challenges.

A2: keep things as they are.

10. I usually …

A1: inspire confidence.

A2: look to others for confidence.

11. I usually …

A1: let my moods and emotions influence my behavior.

A2: have control over my impulses and emotional eruptions.

12. Pressure generally …

A1: causes me to get distracted.

A2: doesn't prevent me from thinking clearly and staying focused.

13. I always …

A1: do what I say that I will.

A2: do what I must and nothing or little more.

14. The trust of others …

A1: is usually just handed to me.

A2: has to be earned through honesty and integrity.

15. I am very often …

A1: flexible in my view of things.

A2: fixed in my vision of events to see them as they are.

16. Facing challenges, I generally ...

A1: work harder and keep up.

A2: manage multiple demands with ease.

17. I always ...

A1: set challenging goals for myself and my team.

A2: achieve lesser goals with less effort.

18. Setback and obstacles generally make me ...

A1: change my expectations or goals.

A2: stay the course and hold my position.

19. Usually, I ...

A1: surpass expectations in achieving my goals.

A2: limit my pursuits to goals I can easily achieve.

20. In the face of opportunities, I am often ...

A1: uncertain about pursuing it.

A2: eager to pursue it.

21. Differences within a group are usually ...

A1: the cause of difficulty.

A2: valued and understood.

22. I consider bias and intolerance ...

A1: a chance to challenge those with the bias.

A2: a thing to ignore so I can get on with my life.

23. I like to help if it's best for ...

A1: completing an important task.

A2: helping others with their thoughts or feelings.

24. I always ...

A1: listen carefully.

A2: listen well enough and read facial cues or body language.

25. The perspectives of others are often ...

A1: clear and well-received.

A2: confusing and unproductive.

26. I typically find social networks ...

A1: a distraction.

A2: a helpful tool.

27. I like to ...

A1: give my customers whatever they ask for.

A2: understand my customer's needs and use my expertise to match the right products or services.

28. I usually …

A1: serve as an advisor.

A2: confirm the customer's opinions or tastes.

29. Customer loyalty and satisfaction …

A1: is central to my work ethic.

A2: is just a cliché and means little to nothing in the final analysis.

30. I always …

A1: inform people of my expectations.

A2: demonstrate the same behavior I expect.

31. I assign projects to workers who …

A1: can do the job well.

A2: will develop and grow with the challenge.

32. I win people over …

A1: with ease.

A2: with difficulty.

32. I always …

A1: follow the changes dictated by others.

A2: suggest changes of my own.

32. I handle difficult people …

A1: with diplomacy.

A2: with frankness.

34. I seek relationships which ...

A1: will help me.

A2: will help us both.

35. My focus is usually ...

A1: stronger on tasks.

A2: stronger on relationships.

Hope you did well. If not, don't fear, as you can always improve your skills and take the test again. That's why it's here, and why *you're* here. Now let's turn our cognitive abilities toward the subject of, well, cognitive abilities.

III

SECTION 3: COGNITIVE ABILITIES

7

OUR PARENTS HELPED US DEVELOP IT, WE'RE NOW OLD ENOUGH TO DEVELOP IT OURSELVES

W e've looked at emotional intelligence, but being truly emotionally intelligent requires cognitive abilities, and being a true leader definitely does. Cognitive abilities occur in the brain; listening, attention, perception. Being attentive to them is crucial for your success.

Cognitive abilities are important in every facet of your life, particularly in the way you interact with others.

Cognitive abilities naturally occur, processing information, recognizing patterns and analyzing problems.

There are different types of cognitive ability. Knowing one from another will be invaluable to your ability to wisely use them all at the proper time and place.

Attention is the way in which you process current information. Paying close attention and retaining what you've learned is perhaps the central cognitive ability. It requires focus and has a direct effect on memory. If you don't absorb it, you won't remember it. On the other hand, the more you absorb, the more you'll retain.

Attention deficit is often a challenge especially in cases of attention deficit/hyperactivity disorder (ADHD). Otherwise, it may strike most people who are multi-tasking or stressed.

There are actually three kinds of attention. Sustained attention is used on a single task over long periods of time. It's central to accomplishing long-term goals. Selective attention is used when there are distractions which are ignored as a matter of discipline. Divided attention is common in this day and age. This is the methodology of the multi-tasker, though it's well-known to be less effective.

Another cognitive ability is memory, the ability to recall information which you have retained. There is short-term memory, things of lesser importance which happened recently, and long-term memory, more important memories from further in the past. Time can often affect the clarity of long-term memories.

Logic and reasoning are cognitive abilities related to problem assessment and solution finding. Memory looks backward, logic and reasoning look to the present and the future.

Auditory and visual processing is all about interpreting information like letters and symbols. It's a useful skill in visualizing goals and outcomes, or for following a map and doing mathematical equations.

Higher cognitive ability generally allows these things to be done quicker. In fact, the higher one's cognitive ability, the faster such mental tasks are generally achieved.

You may not think mathematical skills are as crucial as they once were, and you may be right. But cognitive processing skills may come up in other contexts. Job interviews may require you to assess a hypothetical situation, look ahead to an uncertain and unexpected circumstance, just as will happen in life. Often, you'll be presented with riddles and conundrums which require this cognitive skill set.

Understanding material is important for obvious reasons.

Recognizing patterns of events is central to cognitive ability and one of its most valuable results. If you can see patterns of events, you can predict what will happen. You already know some people may be triggers for others, and you know Mondays are more stressful at the office, so you'll be able to schedule your meetings or manage them accordingly. You'll also be able to gage career opportunities, pitfalls, any number of events others will miss and perhaps fall victim to.

To analyze problems and find options is one of the advanced cognitive abilities. Unexpected things will come up, and options will be necessary. Your job as true leader is to find them, and cognitive ability is the only way you're going to do it.

Brainstorming is hallmark cognitive ability. It's a creative exercise, and it's also often necessary to overcome unexpected obstacles. It's a team activity and good for exciting your team members. It encourages a healthy workplace climate.

Focused attention is key, as we've mentioned. Stay focused and your team will follow your example. This will also help you prioritize and that will make you and your team more efficient and therefor more productive.

IMPROVING YOUR COGNITIVE ABILITY

Like your emotional intelligence, your cognitive ability can be developed and improved. You may not be able to raise your IQ, you can improve your control of this skillset and increase your cognitive ability. Some will be familiar, and with good reason.

Physical activity improves hormone function, and that enhances memory, focus, and retention. It's also good for hand-eye co-ordination and motor skills.

New challenges keep the brain excited and active. Your cognitive ability is like a muscle, and it can atrophy if not worked regularly. New activities almost always include some small failures, which keeps one emotionally aligned not to overthink and to externalize failure from effort. New activities keep brains curious, focused, open to retaining new information, all pillars of cognitive and emotional intelligence.

Brain games are designed specifically to keep your cognitive abilities sharp. They use different abilities, they rely on visual and mathematical patterns, and they can be kind of fun. Just a few minutes a day can vastly improve anyone's cognitive abilities.

Getting enough sleep is crucial to sharpening cognitive abilities. That means less eating and drinking, no cigarettes. Sleep allows your brain to repair and refresh. It may require meditation for some, sleep aids for others.

Keep stress to a minimum in order to maximize cognitive skills. Stress is distractive and reduces focus and hampers attention, retention, and memory. Meditation is great for that.

MEMORY AND MEMORY LOSS

A little more about memory before we move on. We've talked about short-term and long-term memory, but let's look at this a bit more.

The three stages of memory production are:

- *Memory creation* (the result of attention)
- *Memory consolidation* (an organizing and prioritizing of memories)
- *Memory recall* (based on consolidation)

Memory loss can be caused by genetics or personal behavior. Whatever the cause, the brain does have the ability to change in certain ways in a process called *neuroplasticity.* This allows our brains to create new neural pathways to change certain existing connections. The short of it is that memory can be improved, and here's how. They'll be familiar and that's only natural.

Learning something new is the perfect way to improve memory because most things require memory. Languages, artistic skills, just about any new activity will require at least some short-term memory. Using it is the best way to keep from losing it.

Take time for quiet reflection, meditate. It clears away the distractions which challenge memory at just about every stage.

Use your senses in creating memories. The way things smell, touch, and taste makes a big impression on us, so relate events to sensory experiences of that event and this will imprint it on your memory with greater indelibility.

Associate new information with information you already know. One memory will piggie-back on the other.

Summarize what you need to remember from your own perspective. Make it your own and you'll have an easier time remembering it.

Reviewing information is a good way to imprint it on your memory too. Read it and then read it again, then again. Engrain it into your memory.

Mnemonic devices are a great way to increase your memory. Just associate one thing you don't know with something you do know, an exercise we've already visited. For example, if you've never come across the term mnemonic and can't remember it, you might think, *"Use mnemonic or be moronic,"* or something like that.

Seek out challenges, build on your skills, make sure this pursuit has its rewards. It will both inspire and reward your creative mind and stimulate your memory because you'll remember the reward.

Limit screen time to one hour at night. The artificial light isn't good for your sleeping patterns. If you have to read, read from a page with adequate room light. Avoid caffeine at night, as it interrupts healthy sleep patterns.

Relationships are important to brain health too. They encourage brain exercise, empathy, everything we've talked about in this book.

Avoiding stress is good for every part of your life, and your memory will improve for a variety of reasons once you've reduced stress in your life. Stress triggers forgetfulness, for example.

Some ways for managing stress in the workplace may include taking adequate breaks, setting boundaries and expectations, expressing thoughts and feelings, and avoiding multi-tasking.

APPLYING COGNITIVE SKILLS EVERYWHERE

As we've seen, all of these cognitive skills are applicable in every facet of your life. Let's take a look at some concrete examples.

Sustained attention, focusing on single tasks for long periods, is vital in the workplace. You'll use this in the workplace on single task after task, so this cognitive skill is invaluable. But you'll also need it at home, when dealing with long-term tasks like your child's education, home improvements, debt repayment. In social circles, sustained attention is useful in developing and maintaining enduring relationships.

Selective attention, which is trained to avoid distractions, is vital in the workplace, where distractions are everywhere. Every desk has a computer, and that means the internet, one of the greatest sources of distraction in history. There are also phone calls, emergencies, crises of various sorts. Office romances, either coming together or falling apart; the workplace demands selective attention like virtually nowhere else. But the home requires it too. You'll have to muddle through a slew of schoolyard gossip, little conflicts which come and go, and all the same media distractions you get at work. Socially, selective attention allows you to focus on the relationships that matter and ignore the things which don't; loud music, flashing lights, distractions of the social world.

Divided attention is necessary in the workplace, where several projects in different stages of development may need attention at the same time. At home, this can be the needs of a child or more than one, a spouse, perhaps the needs of siblings or the house itself. Electrical, plumbing, foundational issues and more can make homeowning a litany of complex and expensive distractions. You'll often have to keep track of one or more at once, and that's just the house. Throw in the needs of the people in the house and perhaps a few animals and you've got truly divided attention.

Long-term memory is central to the workplace. Lessons from old failures may come into play with new projects, clients from the past may return. At home, long-term memory will keep you from forgetting your wedding anniversary. Socially, long-term memory helps you engage more closely with your long-term friends. Your memories of their lives will be greatly appreciated.

Short-term (or working) memory is vital to organization at the workplace. Deadlines need to be kept in mind. The leader of a team has to have a working knowledge of what each team member is doing, and that requires short-term memory. But household organization is just as vital, and short-term memory will keep you from forgetting the date of your kid's school presentation, your dental appointment. Socially, short-term memory keeps you from missing a lunch date with a friend or the address or directions to the home of a new friend.

Logic and reasoning skills will help you on a daily basis in the workplace. Crises will arise which need quick resolution. Things which were planned can go awry and need to be rethought. A timetable may have to be recalculated due to an unexpected occurrence. At home, logic and reasoning are central to settling disputes (if you have kids, you'll know how valuable this is) and resolving unexpected crises. When somebody drives their car into your living room, you'll know what I mean. Socially, logic and reasoning skills will prevent you from hounding a person who may not be interested in you.

Auditory processing, like visual processing, occur in our lives all day, every day. Even when you're sleeping you may be processing auditory information. At work, this will include important information about ongoing projects, meeting schedules, and unimportant information like office gossip. At home you'll hear a lot of gossip too, but you'll also hear important information about the upkeep of the household and big events in the family's lives. In your social life, you'll hear even more gossip, and that's a good way to tell if you're socializing with the right people. With romances, you'll be hearing details about their lives and tastes and you'll want to remember those. That won't go unnoticed or unrewarded, I promise you.

Visual processing is a bit more interpretive and less direct, which makes proper processing skills even more important. At work, visual processing will be helpful during presentations, which are increasingly relied upon in the corporate world. You'll rely on it to read body language, which tells you a lot about your team, your supervisor, even yourself. While some people learn better from auditory sources and some absorb more from visual stimuli, in the workplace you have to be strong at both. At home, visual processing will tell you how your children are doing. Their body language will tell you if they're happy or stressed. This will be true for your spouse as well. There may be all kinds of visual cues to problems your spouse has never and may never mention. And saying that they never told you there was a problem will not get you off the hook. They shouldn't have had to mention it, and to a large degree they're right. You should have known. Social interaction is much the same. Pay attention to visual cues to ascertain your friends' moods or wellbeing.

Processing speed, which increases along with intelligence, will help you in the workplace by allowing you to solve problems faster and with superior results. This will naturally result in promotion and greater socialization. It will also create better results for the team, and that should create a healthier work climate. At home, decisive problem-solving prevents resentments or other negative feelings to build up among children or spouses. Socially, you'll be able to settle problems between your friends or between them and yourself should they arise. There will be times when quick thinking and measured action are required, perhaps to prevent a bar fight. Friendships can be complicated and may entail all manner of conflicting feelings and hidden resentments.

Cognitive abilities tests generally cover various topics; numerical, verbal, logic, and mechanical reasoning, and spatial awareness.

8

DEEPENING YOUR COGNITIVE ABILITIES

IT STARTS WITH YOUR BODY

W e've briefly touched on the effects of diet and sleep on cognitive abilities, and it only makes sense. Garbage in, garbage out, as they say. But is it true that there are so-called *smart foods* which can actually make you smarter?

Strawberries, blackberries, and blueberries contain flavonoids and anthocyanins, powerful antioxidants which can boost your health overall and your brain health in particular. Studies have shown that they slow cognitive decline.

Dark chocolate has a flavanol also found in berries, tea, cocoa, and various fruits and is beneficial to cognitive processing speed.

Nuts are good for brain health overall, and walnuts are high in alpha-linolenic acid (ALA), an omega-3 fatty acid and linked to higher adult cognitive performances.

Broccoli and other cruciferous vegetables contain sulforaphane, which may protect the brain, and vitamin K. Vitamin K deficiency has been linked to Alzheimer's disease.

Concord grapes, available only for a brief season annually, there is concord grape juice readily available. These big, dark grapes have proven beneficial effects on memory function.

The brain is the body's most fatty organ, so it requires good, omega-3 fats found in salmon, trout, mackerel, sardines, herring, and tuna. Omega-3 deficiency has been associated with Alzheimer's Disease.

Eggs provide choline, essential for good metabolism and is associated with better cognitive test scores in controlled studies.

Seeds in general and pumpkin seeds in particular are great brain food due to the abundance of ALA omega-3's. Pumpkin seeds are high in zinc, vital for optimal brain functioning.

Extracts of the herb sage may have a positive effect on mood and memory, attention and even executive function.

Milk provides the nutrient choline, important for optimal brain health. It also has a big effect on brain development in infants. It may also protect against type 2 diabetes and insulin resistance.

Turmeric is all the rage these days, and for good reason. It's great for heartburn, gas, and other digestive issues. It's a great anti-inflammatory too.

Cocoa powder is also packed with flavonoids, particularly epicatechin, which appears to improve cognition and may also treat or even prevent diabetes.

Leafy, green kale has an abundance of the mineral called *manganese*, and also a ton of vitamins A, C, and K.

Beets are high in nitrates, which relax blood vessels and increase circulation, particularly to the brain.

Olive oil is central to the so-called *Mediterranean diet.* It's high in polyphenols, which have been proven to lower risk of Parkinson's and Alzheimer's diseases.

Bone broth is high in protein, which the brain needs to function at its best.

Beans are also high in protein, and ALA omega-3s too. Beans are also rich in carbohydrates, and those are turned into glucose which fuels the brain.

Tea may aid weight loss and help prevent cancer, and it has proven benefits for the brain. It's caffeine boosts energy while amino acid L-theanine helps the brain to relax. Green tea in particular is associated with reduced risk of some cognitive disorders.

Beef is rich in iron, which is central to good overall health, as it carries oxygen from the lungs to bodily tissues. Fatigue is a common sign of iron deficiency.

You may never have heard of yerba mate, but it's common in South America as a hot drink. It has 24 minerals and herbs, 15 different amino acids and a variety of polyphenols, plus theophylline and theobromine.

Whole-grain oats are easily converted to glucose, the brain's favored fuel source. Oats also offer B vitamins, magnesium, and iron. And they won't increase your blood sugar.

Lentils have a lot of folate, one of the B vitamins which is shown to increase cognitive performance in controlled studies. B vitamins decreases homocysteine, an amino acid. Excessive amino acids may reduce cognitive ability.

Flaxseeds high levels of ALA may have a strong impact on suffers of Alzheimer's Disease. Ground flaxseed is often sprinkled over a salad, over cold or hot cereal, or blended into a smoothie.

And there are foods and supplements which are proven to reduce stress and anxiety.

A member of the mint family, lemon balm has been studied for anti-anxiety effects. Omega-3 fatty acids reduced anxiety symptoms by 20% in one study. The herb ashwagandha has likewise been proven effective in reducing stress and anxiety symptoms.

The antioxidants found in green tea increase serotonin levels to lower anxiety and stress. The root called valerian contains valerianic acid, which is a powerful sleep aid and alters the GABA (gamma-aminobutyric acid) receptors. This lowers anxiety.

A member of the pepper family, kava kava is used in the South Pacific to treat mild stress and anxiety.

HAVE YOU BEEN STRESSED LATELY? YOU MUST LEARN HOW TO REDUCE IT

We've looked at stress and its effects on the body and the brain. Stress causes inflammation, poor sleeping and eating habits, substance abuse, ensuing weight gain and ill-health, depression, premature death by stroke or heart disease and suicide.

And we've looked at ways to reduce stress, including meditation. Let's take a closer look at good ways to relieve stress.

Exercise, better sleep habits, better nutrition, avoidance of substance abuse, mindful awareness, adapting a growth mindset, time management; all are critical for a more stress-free life. Clearer communications with others will always reduce or may even prevent stress and anxiety.

Meditation is a popular way to relieve stress, and though we've touched on it briefly, a closer look is probably a good idea here.

When you meditate, you sit quietly and still and focus on just one thing. It might be your breath, the steady in-and-out pattern of inhaling and exhaling deeply and slowly. You might focus on a single focal point or on a repeated phrase or mantra. But there's a lot more to it, as there are lots of ways to meditate.

First, meditation can be grouped into two categories. Calming (*samatha*) meditation cultivates a quiet, peaceful state in the manner I just described, by focusing on breathing or a focal point or a mantra.

Insight (*vipassana*) meditation, on the other hand, develops qualities of character such as wisdom and compassion by focusing on the effects of the breath on the body rather than on the breathing itself. You may start with calming meditation and go on to insight meditation later and them combine the two.

There are eight core techniques from Tibetan and Burmese Buddhist traditions. They combine of both insight and calming meditations.

We've already touched on focused attention, which directs the focus on breath, a focal point, or a mantra. If your mind wanders, return it to whatever you're focusing on.

Body scan meditation directs the attention to the body, starting at the bottom and concentrating on each part of the body and how it feels.

Noting is the practice of being aware of both distractions and recentering focus during meditation. It's a kind of focused awareness of these shifts, how they are caused and then controlled. Use this technique in combination with other techniques when you're ready.

Visualization entails conjuring an image in your mind and focusing on that. It may be a visualization of something or someone you desire, the manifestation of a long-term goal like a home of your own.

Loving kindness meditation focuses specifically on people, even on some we don't like. This technique focuses on directing positive energy toward someone who may be a source of negative energy.

The technique of skillful compassion entails putting the focus on a person you love and then focusing on the effects, the way that positive energy affects your body, comparable to facets of body scan meditation.

With the technique of resting awareness, the mind truly rests. It's an advanced technique, built upon a working knowledge of the other techniques we've looked at.

The reflection technique entails asking a question during meditation, such as, *"How can you help others,"* or, *"What things do you have to be grateful for?"* invites you to ask yourself a question: perhaps something such as, "What are you most grateful for?" Be mindful to use you and not I, or you'll be tempted to answer. The reflection technique focuses on the question.

Transcendental meditation focuses on a greater power, whatever your notion of God or a higher power may be.

Those are all self-monitored techniques, but some of the following techniques require a qualified master.

- Yoga meditation often uses Kundalini yoga among other types of yoga and is most effective in a class.
- Chakra meditation focuses on the body's core centers of energy or chakras to keep them open and aligned, remedying various mental and physical symptoms.
- Comparably, the Chinese practice of Qigong meditation harnesses energy by keeping pathways called *meridians* open and aligned.

- Sound bath meditation uses instruments like gongs and bowls to create calming sound vibrations.

BRAIN EXERCISES ARE NOT ONLY FUN, BUT THEY'RE ALSO GOOD FOR YOU

Remember that your mind is like a muscle and it has to be kept in shape. These exercises will go a long way to making your mind stronger, your brain more efficient, and your life better.

Besides the specific tactics you'll learn here are the most common methods of exciting the brain. Board games, new activities, new languages; these are time-tested ways to improve your cognitive powers. Other than that, here are some specific ways you can increase your cognitive abilities.

Here's one great trick to sharpening your memory and increasing your brainpower. Try to draw a map of your neighborhood entirely from memory. Fill in as many of the street names as you can. You won't get all of them, of course, as the likelihood of your knowing every street in your neighborhood is pretty slim. But you will know some of them, the streets around your house and workplace. It's the exercise that counts, not the results.

Are you righthanded? Try favoring your left hand. If you're a lefty, try living as a righty for a full day. Be deliberate about it. Open doors with the other hand, scratch yourself and sign a credit card receipt with the hand you don't normally use. This challenges your brain and your motor-control skills and keeps both sharp.

Test your recall by making lists from memory. Write down what you bought at the supermarket, what exercises you did at the gym and in what order. You might get more specific if you're ready to challenge yourself. Because your task is to memorize that list. Now tend to that task. Memorize as much as you can. You won't remember it all, but remember that it's the exercise that counts, not the results.

Engage in the practice of doing mathematical equations. It's a powerful technique for a variety of purposes, including erectile stamina (you fellas know what I mean). But just the process of running mathematical equations stimulates the brain and keeps it agile.

Here's a fun and challenging mathematical challenge. Pick any 3-digit number then add 3 to that digit three different times. Then subtract 7 from that new number 7 times. For example, you may start with 100. Then add 3 to that three separate times, for a total of 109. Now subtract 7 from that number, and do that seven times. It reduces 109 to 102, then 95 and so on. Remember that you're not filing your taxes, so the results don't matter. It's the exercise that counts.

Create a word picture. You may be thinking of a vision board, which includes pictures of the things you hope to achieve. With this exercise, you simply visualize a word, then think of other words that begin or end with the same letters. *Clouds* may become *cowards* and *sensations*. The results may surprise you.

Try eating new foods. The same old foods put your body into a rut. But new flavors excite your body and your mind. Remember that culinary is one of the arts, and arts stimulate the brain. The culinary arts are unique, as they bring a kind of nourishment and satisfaction that other arts just can't, not even mixology.

Try mixology. There is a lot of data behind the soft science of cocktail creation. Memory and processing are vital, and there's instant satisfaction to your efforts. Those may actually inhibit your memory later, but nothing's free, right?

Hobbies like drawing, knitting, painting, or puzzles are a great way to keep the mind sharp and even increase cognitive skills. A new sport or physical activity will have the same effect, as we've discussed. Fencing is a good choice, or the martial arts. Both are rooted in philosophy and rules of engagement which may overlap into various other facets of your life. Yoga and meditation are popular and beneficial in any number of ways.

Try showering with your eyes closed. You'll be using your tactile senses of touch to feel the shampoo and soaps and the like. Your memory of the shower will guide your hand to the controls. But be careful with this exercise. Be cautious of slippage or of setting the water temperature!

Change your routine. Feel free to create new routines if you need them to get along, and a lot of people do. But change things up. Variety will keep your mind engaged even in the simplest tasks.

Turn things upside down. No, I don't mean that figuratively. You're used to seeing things a certain way, and this can create mental lethargy. Do you have an alarm clock? Turn it upside down literally. Your brain will be able to understand what numbers it's really looking at, and putting it through that exercise will only strengthen your cognitive ability. Is there a vase on the dining room table, flip it over. It may not seem like a lot, but do it enough and your eye and then your brain will be drawn to it.

Switch seats at the table. If it's a conference room table or the dinner table or even a seat in a classroom, we tend to find a spot and stick to it. But switching things around helps you to see things from a different perspective, from another person's perspective, and that strengthens empathy and a number of other cornerstones of emotional intelligence.

Aroma therapy is a powerful technique. The olfactory senses are closest to the brain and therefore, have the most powerful effects. If you doubt that, consider this; do you remember what your childhood living room smelled like? Your father's cigar tobacco or your mother's favored cleaning products? Think of the smell of bacon. 'Nough said.

Drive with the window down. Well, in this case you'd be better served to be the passenger, but it works while you're driving too. This is a powerful exercise because the hippocampus, which is the area of the brain which processes memories, is also associated with sounds, odors, sights. So, take a drive and try to identify the smells you pass; freshly cut grass, a fish cannery, a chicken ranch. Savor and be grateful and experience those smells, bad or good.

Try this; fill a cup full of change. Then swish the change around in the cup and try to imagine the value of the change. Concentrate on the weight, the sound, the sensory input. Try to guess the value. Again, you may not succeed, but it's not a midway game, it's a brain exercise and it should have terrific benefits.

Read aloud. It may sound silly and childish, but it's really not as easy as it sounds. Literate and intelligent people find it hard to read aloud. The sound of one's voice is distracting, the impression it may make causes insecurity, and the twin chores of reading and speaking can be surprisingly challenging. Try it right now by reading this paragraph. Go ahead, I'll wait. Now, did it sound the same as when you were reading it silently? When it does, your cognitive abilities will have been improved!

Make a list of random words, then see if you can remember them. Make sure they're random; waistcoat, sucker punch, burning man, cucumber. The longer the list, the more challenging and the better your performance and the better your benefits.

Imagine a crossword puzzle. It's a series of squares, some in lines and others up against one another. Not count the squares, but not just the individual squares; include the squares created by four or more squares in a cluster. How many squares are there?

Here's one for the left brain. Take the word WALL and change one letter at a time until you get to the word FIRM. The trick is that every change has to create an actual word. For example, you can change WALL into WILL, then WILL into FILL. Once you've completed this challenge, try it again with the same word and a different word. Turning FIRM back into WALL won't be much of a challenge. Turn FIRM into COAT instead. It can be done. Do it. Then pick other four-word or even five-word challenges. Keep doing it, make it a hobby.

Try this: Arrange three toothpicks into the letter nine. Don't bend or break any of them. Can you do it? Hey, it's not supposed to be easy, it's supposed to be a challenge!

Here's a powerful technique: Write a cluster of letters and numbers on a piece of paper, but allow significant space between them. Start at 1 and draw a line to the nearest letter A. Proceed from there to the number 2 and draw a line from there to the letter B. B leads you to 3 which leads you to C, and so forth.

You might try this exercise: Look at the words below and rearrange the letters of each to create words for common colors. Only one of them is a primary color.

- ENOLYL
- RAIGET
- LEWRE
- OVGOEN

What did you come up with? Keep trying, or observe your results.

The proverb experiment is always challenging and helpful. Below is a proverb with all the vowels removed. Just insert the right vowels to complete the proverb. It's like *Wheel of Fortune* in your own home, and your prize is greater cognitive strength.

- TWH
- DSRB
- TTRT
- HNN

Hey, it's not supposed to be easy!

Here's another fun word scramble challenge. How many words can you create from these letters? OGEUNRY

Here's a riddle to excite your mind and keep your cognitive skills alive:

Frank has eccentric tastes; a fan of football but not of rugby; he loves beer but he hates ale; Frank drives a Ferrari though he won't drive a Lamborghini. Keeping these things in mind, is finicky Frank more likely to prefer cycling or skiing?

Try eating with chopsticks. It involves motor control and creates instant gratification.

Now that we've looked into some practical, applicable ways to boost our emotional and cognitive skills, let's take a closer look at crucial thinking; it's central to both and key to your success as a true leader.

IV

DEVELOP YOUR CRITICAL THINKING SKILLS AND USE THEM

9

WHY CRITICAL THINKING SKILLS?

C ritical thinking emphasizes analysis and interpretation. Roughly put, it's not the facts which truly matter, but their evaluation. It's a disciplined process of conceptualizing, analyzing, applying, synthesizing, and evaluating information. This information is generated by or gathered from experience, observation, reasoning, reflection, and communication.

Put more simply, critical thinking allows you to understand things more clearly and make wiser choices or beliefs.

Critical thinking isn't everyday thinking, which is often automatic. Critical thinking is deliberate. Without critical thinking, a person may fall into bad mental habits such as the ones described below.

Ignorant certainty, for example, is the certainty that every question has a single correct answer. But this is often not the case in day-to-day life. This is a fixed mindset where a growth mindset would better serve everyone involved, the thinker in particular.

Naive relativism is like the flipside of ignorant certainty, the belief that all arguments are equal and that there is no single truth or right answer to any question.

But with adequate critical thinking, one may enjoy several distinct benefits.

Critical thinking allows the formation of opinions and having intelligent conversations. It's crucial for self-evaluation. It's critical for decision-making and exploitation avoidance in every facet of your life.

Those who think critically tend to comprehend the connections between ideas, prioritize ideas and arguments, manage arguments, recognize errors of reasoning, handle problems in a systematic and consistent manner, and reflect on their own assumptions, values, and beliefs.

CRITICAL THINKING SKILLS

Those who have these sharp critical thinking skills are well-prepared to deal with almost any critical thinking challenge. Ask yourself if these aren't areas that you could improve in your own critical thinking.

Critical thinkers gather Information. Do you, or do you just wing it? Critical thinkers are observant, they pay attention to the smallest details. Do you, or do you not gloss over the little stuff? There's a lot of information out there, so don't feel badly if you miss small things, then develop that part of your critical thinking.

Critical thinkers infer, use reason and logic for creative problem-solving. They can rationalize, or apply reason to a situation. Reason generally includes either induction (direct information), deduction (indirect information leading to a conclusion), or analogy (using comparisons and previous experience).

They reflect to recalibrate their perspective and make relaxed decisions. They create even if they're not artistically creative. Critical thinkers create solutions, new approaches, insightful analyses. Do you reflect and let that feed your creativity? Or is it always pedal-to-the-medal.

Critical thinking requires organization enough to classify and sequence, or to group and order ideas or items according to shared characteristics. They compare and contrast to similar situations or circumstances. Are you as quick to organize and compartmentalize? Do you keep past lessons or information in mind?

Critical thinkers consider cause and effect and utilize foresight. Do you, or do you just hope it works out?

Critical thinkers synthesize different approaches and ideas to form new ones. Do you, or do you not just apply the usual remedies? Critical thinkers also brainstorm. Do you, or do you not just go with the first idea that pops into your head. A lot of people will say the first idea is probably the best idea and cite overthinking as a reason to go with the gut. Do you? Remember, think for yourself.

Critical thinkers prioritize to keep crises in perspective. Do you, or is every crisis the end of the world? Drama is not part of critical thinking.

Critical thinkers also summarize to ensure a thorough understanding of the event or situation. Do you keep records of these events, journals? Maybe you should.

These skills work great in combination too, like most of what we're discussing in this book. There's a lot of overlap, and something learned in one field of study connects to another.

We mentioned a critical thinking cycle before, let's take a closer look at that. The stages usually occur in order, one following the other. The cycle begins with observation of information or notes experimental results.

Observation is followed by feeling, an intellectual reaction to the new input. This leads to wondering, plumbing the causes or processes of an event. People wonder about who, what, where, when, why, and how, among other things.

Imagining follows wondering, turning wondering away from the past (the circumstances of the cause) toward the future.

Inference follows imagining and visualizes results. Also looking to the future, imagining adds to wondering the question *What if?*

Knowledge is (hopefully) the result of imagining and inference. Knowledge comes from research into previous data to answer the question *What if?*

Experimenting follows knowledge and represents the application of the knowledge attained.

Consulting on the results of the experiment follows and is crucial to the critical thinking cycle.

Consultations may lead to analyzing and identifying arguments, when consultations may be challenged or alternatives considered. Question and understand the source of the arguments and their purpose in every case.

In the judging stage of the critical thinking cycle, one makes a judgment based on the analysis of the arguments.

The final stage is deciding, wherein a choice is made and a plan of action set about to move forward.

SEVEN WAYS TO THINK CRITICALLY

Here are seven ways you can think more critically, starting right here and now!

In our increasingly complex world, don't be afraid to ask basic questions. The basics are easy to lose track of and it's vital to always have them in the back of your mind. Remember that there are no stupid questions.

You may also try to question some basic assumptions. It's like asking basic questions, but of yourself and your perspective.

Be mindful of what your common mental processes are. Try to avoid the common mental shortcuts a lot of us take and really focus on what you're thinking, when and why. You might want to keep a thought journal to illustrate the patterns in your mental processes. You might have biases and prejudices which are more glaring in an objective light.

Reversing things is a great way to think critically. De-engineer a problem if you have to, or read something from the bottom up to scan for errors. It challenges the mind and prevents lazy mental shortcuts.

Evaluating existing evidence is a good way to think critically. Learn from previous instances, previous mistakes. Know the data which has already been collected. When you do, question that evidence in terms of who gathered it, how they did that, and why they did it.

Think for yourself, always. Research will guide you, but your efforts may advance that collected knowledge.

Accepting fallibility is another way to think critically. Nobody functions at maximum capacity all the time, not even you. Make allowances for this with yourself and others.

Critical thinking and decision making often go hand-in-hand. There are elements of decision-making which go hand-in-hand with critical thinking. Both entail logic, (a direct or indirect connection of causes and events), truth (unbiased data), context (external factors and pressures), and alternatives (potential solutions).

THINKING CRITICALLY IN YOUR PROFESSIONAL & PERSONAL LIFE

Critical thinking in the workplace and the home takes many forms and can improve your career in a number of ways.

Critical thinking brings you to clear goal setting, knowing what you want and how to make it happen. This includes knowing what your team members are capable of and what they're willing to do. This is as true when working on a project like an ad campaign or getting your family through the annual summer season when the kids are off school. If you want the ad campaign done on time, what will be required? To keep the kids active and the house quiet, what should you do?

Foresight is central to critical thinking, and it's often required in the workplace. What if moving a project to a different location would be helpful because the location is more optimal, but the move would sacrifice some of your best team members. Is there some compromise or alternative? It's the same when planning family events or seasons. What if one child is miserable at summer camp? What if one sibling becomes jealous of the birthday gifts given to another? Looking ahead to possible outcomes, or foresight, will lead you to the answer.

Conferring with a mentor is a great way to think critically in the workplace. They should be an authority in your area of specialty and experience which you may lack. This is a prime application of critical thinking and will also strengthen your relationship. For domestic matters, mentorship can be a powerful tool too. Friends who had children before you or have been married longer will have invaluable insights to share.

Team-building games and exercises are a great way to improve a team's ability to think critically. It's helpful for the leader as well, as it gives them a chance to think critically and analyze the team's overall executive functionality and that of its members. Games and exercises are great for the family too, and for the same reasons. You'll also create a healthier climate in both arenas.

CRITICAL THINKING SKILLS WILL REVOLUTIONIZE YOUR DECISION-MAKING ABILITIES WITHIN DAYS...

Critical thinking means asking questions, but that can be an art unto itself. Foresight is required, as are curiosity, noting, mindfulness, a lot of the skills you've already acquired from this book. Here are a few more relating in particular to critical questioning. You'll be asking *who, what, were, when, why, how,* and *what if*, among other things.

Consider these points when you formulate critical questions.

- Good questions are designed with the intent of soliciting specific information. So, it should be stated clearly, concisely, and with direct meaning. Vagueness or subtext should be strictly avoided in critical questioning.
- Frame your questions properly. Put it in the right context, make sure they're not just declarations with question marks.
- Try using open-ended questions (*"How does that make you*

feel?") instead of closed-ended questions that will likely end with a *yes* or *no* (*"Do you feel good?"*).

- Use follow-up questions and keep them open-ended too.
- When you're asking these questions, make sure they're the right questions. To know this, answer a few for yourself first and make sure of a few key points.
- Make sure your purpose is clear, as we said, be specific in order to get the proper specific response. Instead of asking *if*, ask *when*. Instead of when, suggest a time and place and have a backup ready.
- Specific questions have specific purposes; definition (*"What does working hard mean to you?"*), comparative (*"How do we excel?"*), causal (*"If we make this move, what are the benefits and drawbacks?"*) and evaluative (*"What's working and what isn't?"*).

PROBLEM-SOLVING MODELS

There are various problem-solving models, each with their own specific construct. Let's take a closer look at some of the most effectual.

The simple *6-Step Problem Solving* includes these easy-to-understand problem-solving steps:

Objective-finding to identify the problem and begin finding the solution. Fact-finding collects data, problem-finding analyzes the data, idea-finding brainstorms based on the problem and the data. Solution-finding settles on a new plan of action, and acceptance-finding moves on from that solution.

Additionally, these six come in three phases of problem solving. These are exploring the challenge (Objective- and fact-finding), generating ideas (problem- and idea-finding) and preparing for action (solution- and accepting finding).

The Yale version of the Soft Stage Management model (SSM), uses six steps of action for problem solving, once again in order (most of these models observe an order to the steps or stages).

First one defines the problem, then determines the root cause, then develops alternative solutions, selects one of those and implements it, then evaluates the outcome.

Large group decisions, long-term restructuring, and comparative decision-making benefit from this model.

The political economic social technological model (PEST) is widely used for decision-making and includes, as you might have guessed, consideration of political, economic, social, and technological influences on any decision-making. It's a powerful tool for evaluating markets or strategies or managing large-scale change.

A SWOT model analysis includes focus on strengths, weaknesses, opportunities, and threats. It's effective for identifying toxic or faulty processes or behaviors fast and it's beneficial to brainstorming and strategy building, as well as gathering and organizing information.

As one of the first systematic techniques for observing organizations' weaknesses, the Failure Mode and Effects Analysis (FMEA) system often is used as a diagnostic tool for companies and other large groups. FMEA analyzes the elements of failure and its effects in order to correct them in the present and prevent them in the future. It's widely used in manufacturing and assembly lines. Henry Ford was an early proponent!

Another anagram-based model is the CATWOE defines six areas where soft system problems arise. They include clients, actors, transformation, worldview, owner, and environment and focuses the discussion of those items in regard to potential actions. It's effective for identifying problems, implementing solutions, as well as organizing and then aligning various goals.

A cause and effect analysis, known as *Fishbone* or *Ishikawa diagrams,* takes four steps into account when assessing a single effect to find potential causes. The four steps include identifying a problem, working out which are the involved factors, identifying potential causes, and analyzing a diagram to get ready for action. Categorization and compartmentalization are key to discover proper causes and to understand their effects.

If you're in manufacturing, you might use the six M model (which includes method, material, man power, measurement, mother nature). Those in the service industry often use the five S model (which includes surroundings, suppliers, systems, skills, safety).

CRITICAL THINKING TEST

Try this critical thinking test and see if you can shore up your critical thinking skills! The answers are included in a second set just below the questions:

1) You have two jugs, one an eight-gallon and the other a three-gallon jug, both unmarked. You need precisely four gallons of water. Assuming there's a nearby faucet, how do you get the water?

2) What amount can be added to 1,000,000 such that the sum will be higher than if you multiplied it by the same amount?

3) Find the two one-word answers to this riddle:

The floor of a boat or ship,

you walk on me when at sea;

Make the C an S,

At school, you may sit on me.

I am which two things?

4) A man tells the press he's quitting his job due to, "Illness and fatigue." It's neither precisely a lie nor the truth. Why did he quit his job?

5) Find the two one-word answers to this riddle.

A pseudonym for sick,

The forehead is hot;

Insert an H in the front,

Still, a mountain, I'm surely not.

I am which two things?

6) Solve this riddle:

A goose, a duck, a horse, and a goat walk into a barn at different times. The first is a mammal. The duck precedes the goose and the goose preceded the horse. Which entered first?

7) A woman goes to bed one summer night and woke up in the middle of winter. How can this be so?

Here are the answers:

1) Fill the three-gallon container three times, dumping each load into the eight-gallon container. On the third time, there will be one gallon left in the three-gallon container. Empty the eight-gallon container and pour the single gallon from the smaller container into the larger. Then fill the three-gallon container, add it to the single gallon in the larger container, for a sum total of four gallons.

2) zero, or any negative or fraction less than one.

3) Deck and desk

4) The coach of a professional ball team, he was "sick and tired" of his team's weak performances.

5) Ill and hill.

6) the first to enter was the goat.

7) She was on a ship which passed the equator line while she was sleeping.

How'd you do? Some were easier than others, right?

Now let's take a look at social skills, at the heart of both critical thinking and emotional intelligence.

V

BUILDING BETTER RELATIONSHIPS, THRIVING IN YOUR CHOSEN PATH, & BECOMING THE BEST LEADER THAT YOU CAN BE

SOCIAL SKILLS

W e use social skills to interact and communicate, verbally and also non-verbally utilizing body language, gestures, and personal appearance. We're social creatures, after all, so social communication is not only natural but necessary.

When we speak, body language and tone of voice has great effect on how that message comes across Knowing this and managing it properly is at the heart of social skills.

But as it is with all skillsets, such as leadership skills, emotional intelligence, and cognitive ability, social skills can be learned and improved. So, if you feel your social skills need work, let's get to it. There's not a moment to spare.

Advantages to sharper social skills include better relations and more of them, better communications in business and other aspects of your personal life, greater efficiency, better career opportunities and projects, increased happiness overall.

Social skills share a certain set of characteristics. For example, social skills are basically goal-directed. They are usually appropriate to the circumstance, and different social skills are best used in different social situations.

Greater social skills are invaluable in your career. A lot of networking takes place outside of the office, after all. Conferences, lunch meetings, dinners, they all skirt the line between work and social arenas. Some career benefits to stronger social skills include gathering ideas, techniques, information, and perspectives, freely providing perspective, collaborating with others and accomplishing shared goals, providing mutual support, expanding your network, and gaining honest feedback.

In the office, better social skills will also encourage interactivity, creativity, efficiency, and a healthier work climate. And since the workplace is such a communication-heavy environment, with phone calls and emails and meetings and other things, social skills are all the more important.

In addition to the aforementioned effective communication skills, good social skills in the workplace will aid with conflict resolution between team members (or even between you and a team member) and thereby encourage active listening, which is key to conflict resolution. Your good example of social skills will lead your team to adopt the same.

Empathy, another familiar concept to us from previous information in this book, and it's central to any set of social skills. Without it, there can be few real connections in either social, professional, or familial areas of your life. It's as potent in the workplace as anywhere else.

Social skills are strengthened by and also strengthen relationship management, a way to organize the various relationships in your life, and a lot of them may not be yours but between your team members, at home between your children. Still, your social skills will be key to managing those relationships.

Social skills both provide and engender respect, and this is crucial when you're a true leader in the workplace or at home or out with the gang.

The ways to improve your social skills are comparable to the remedies to emotional ignorance or lack of true leadership, which probably won't surprise you. They include getting feedback and mentorship, setting goals and encouraging others to share your commitment, identifying resources and areas for improvement or practice.

Body language is especially potent in the workplace. The way you carry yourself will influence how others carry themselves. Slouching and slumping, pointing and yelling, snarling and looking around with shifting eyes and a dubious manner will have corrosive effects. It tells people more about you than anything you could say.

THE CONSEQUENCE OF LACKING SOCIAL SKILLS

To lack social skills is, frankly, to be awkward. Awkwardness is defined roughly as a sort of feeling of social embarrassment, or it's a situation which is not relaxed but difficult. People who are awkward don't know how to communicate clearly, they're withdrawn and generally are not true leaders. They often lack emotional intelligence, about themselves or others. Are you socially awkward? If you are, there are ways to escape it. Let's take a closer look to the betterment of your life in every way, shape, or form. Those who are or feel awkward often feel out of place in almost any situation.

Signs that you may be socially awkward include being avoided by people in social settings and you avoid others in the same way. Dates go poorly and intimate relationships end fairly quickly. Social circles are small and they have an oversized effect on your self-esteem. Over-thinking and worry about others' opinions are common. Being called weird may be common, and hurtful.

Reasons for awkwardness may include childhood influences. An overly aggressive parent or sibling may be the cause, or introverted parents who set the example and were awkward themselves. Poverty may engender adulthood insecurity, or a pattern of romantic rejection. Children who grew up in the last ten years may have spent too much time online, and lacking in personal interaction contributes to their insecurity and awkwardness.

Mental or behavioral disorders may also be to blame. ADHD, various complexes, and autism spectrum disorder are common causes of social awkwardness, as are substance abuse and depression. An outsized admiration for someone can cause it too. Who might not be a little awkward meeting their hero?

But you can correct social awkwardness! You might try developing your confidence, but how do you do that? Well, you can use a lot of techniques we recommend in this and other books. Use the Pomodoro Method to break big tasks down into little tasks with manageable milestones. Try new things to stimulate your brain.

Keep in mind that different situations require different behaviors and be flexible, if you can. Being awkward on a date may come down to simply not knowing what's appropriate. These days, it's hard for almost anyone to tell! Do some research, gather your data and decide on a plan of action.

Accountability has its place too. Those who are awkward often feel that they're more accountable than they are, they can't forgive themselves. They're often of a fixed mindset which tells them they can't change, that they're doomed to lives of isolation.

HABITS THAT WILL IMPROVE NOT ONLY YOUR SOCIAL SKILLS BUT YOUR CURRENT RELATIONSHIPS AS WELL

You have to be mindful of your behavior if you're to improve your social skills, as with any other skill set. Here are some concrete ways you can do just that, and in virtually no time.

We've already talked about being an active listener, so you shouldn't be surprised to see it pop here. Active listening is a potent social skill, to be sure. It gives the other person reason to open up, creates stronger, trust-based bonds, and familiarity will defeat the nervousness of the unknown which contributes to awkwardness.

Some people do better one-on-one, others thrive in a big crowd. Perhaps counterintuitively, those who are awkward are often more comfortable in a crowd, where they can feel lost and invisible. Others are intimidated by big crowds and aren't sure how to react.

Avoid negativity and complaining, two big factors to creating an awkward situation even if you don't consider yourself personally awkward. It's a drag anyway, so stop it.

Remembering people's names not only reduces awkwardness, but forgetting their names creates incredible awkwardness all on its own. Use a mnemonic device to imprint the name in your brain. It's such an impressive and rare skill, anybody would be impressed. It demonstrates focus, active listening, empathy, all hallmarks of cognitive ability, emotional intelligence, and true leadership. Likewise, remember their stories. It will make an even bigger and better impression for all the same reasons.

Resist the urge to talk too much. Don't mind the lull and feel you have to constantly keep a conversation going. It's a sure sign of insecurity, and that is a chief generator of social awkwardness. Let the conversation recharge, there's nothing wrong with that. Maybe the other person will start blathering, and their social awkwardness will make you seem all the more cool and collected.

Following up is a good way to defeat awkwardness. It's often uncomfortable to see someone you never called back, and not knowing their disposition only increases nervousness and awkwardness.

Always know when to make an exit. Don't linger. It's a sign of insecurity. And the more you talk, the greater a chance you'll say the wrong thing and stumble into an awkwardness sand trap which you may not be able to dig yourself out of. You can't really have that much to say anyway. Observe the old showbiz adage and leave 'em wanting more.

Love is the greatest social skill, so show it. Whatever you love, share that. It will give you strength, reasserting and reenforcing your sense of self. It's also a great way to open up, and familiarity defeats awkwardness.

YOUR FACIAL EXPRESSIONS SPEAK FOR YOU

Find your so-called *resting face*. It's not easy, because we're all trained to put on a brave face, to change our behavior, even this article recommends mindful smiling. But you should make efforts to be comfortable behind your own face without smiling, without frowning, without any emotion at all. There will be times when you're not emotional, after all. What do you look like then? Whatever it is, the more comfortable you are with it, the more comfortable you'll be with yourself and others. Teeth-grinding and/or jaw-clenching (called *bruxism*) wrinkles, and other dangerous or unflattering results are likely otherwise.

Research by the National Institute of Dental and Craniofacial Research indicates that over 10 million Americans suffer from TMJ syndrome, or temporomandibular joint dysfunction syndrome. Practice various muscle relaxation techniques, meditate, and be mindful of your body language.

Make eye contact more often, but don't be aggressive about it. Do it until it feels good, then don't be afraid to back off a bit. That will draw their eye contact to you to reconnect, and set the intimate example. Cultural differences will affect eye contact, naturally, as some cultures find it disrespectful and a challenge to authority.

Smiling more often is proven to have beneficial effects on a person's overall outlook. The act itself is associated with dopamine and serotonin, a mood-stabilizing hormone. It's also a proven phone sales and tech support line technique, as the shape of your mouth affects the tone of the voice. You'll also be creating a healthier social climate, and that will alleviate stress and reduce awkwardness.

Be mindful of hand gestures and gesticulation. It can open you up and relax you, but some hand movements, such as tucking hands into pockets or wringing your fingers, are sure signs of insecurity and awkwardness.

Remember that a firm handshake not only engenders respect but it generates confidence. Keep a paper towel in your pocket if you've got clammy palms.

SOCIAL SKILLS & CHARISMA ARE THE KEYS TO BEING SEEN AS MORE THAN JUST THE 'BOSS' OR 'MANAGER' BY THOSE YOU LEAD

Charisma might be thought of as the opposite of awkwardness. It's a certain charm, an attractiveness. People with charisma have an influence over those around them. They're often confident because they're better educated or more skilled than others.

There are two distinct types of charismatic people. Some are quiet but beguiling, relying on glances or physical beauty or sheer mystique for their charisma. Others are passionate communicators, they might be inspirational speakers, comics, singers, or actors.

Affability is a constant in either case. Those who have charisma are approachable, even if they're not extroverted.

Try rating your own charisma on a scale from one to five (five being the most positive) in terms of these statements.

I am a person who...

> *... has a significant presence in a room with others*
> *... can influence people*
> *... can lead a group*
> *... comforts others*
> *... smiles often*
> *... gets along with almost anyone*

Now add up the total and divide by six, and that's your average score. If you rated higher than 4, you're ahead of most.

Certain skills comprise and contribute this affability and influence. Developing influence (through presence, ability to lead and to influence); being confident in a variety of situations, either one-on-one or in a group, either as a leader or team member; they're optimistic and positive; charismatic people are persuasive and influential.

The charismatic will open up emotionally but in a measured fashion, never complaining. They are interest*ing* and interest*ed*.

Charismatic people are often engaging, good storytelling, witty, but they don't seek to dominate any conversation. They know the value of the lull, as it demonstrates security and confidence. They laugh at others' jokes and are free with their compliments.

The charismatic are empathetic and engender trust.

Charismatic people communicate clearly. They don't mumble and mutter. So, take some time to work on your speaking voice. It's your most effective method of communication, after all. Make the most of it. Shift it downward deeper into your chest. It may take some practice or some lessons, but you may find it very worthwhile. From trial lawyers to drill sergeants, the voice is a powerful instrument for charisma and influence, which is a big part of charisma as we've already seen.

CHARISMATIC LEADERS

Charismatic leaders are necessary to our societies all over the world. They lead movements and fight for others, for a better world. They lead with courage and conviction. They also lead with compassion for their team members and for their needs and desires.

Charismatic leaders often arise in times of crisis. They lead their followers with a deep sense of purpose and passion. Some of the great leaders in history have been charismatic leaders, including Winston Churchill, Ronald Reagan, Mahatma Gandhi, Dr. Martin Luther King, Jr, Malcom X, and many others.

On the other hand, some of history's worst and most reviled leaders have been equally charismatic, including Adolph Hitler, Joseph Stalin, and Vladimir Putin.

Charismatic leaders are often inspirational and influential to those around them, they're often growth-minded, companies led by such people are often moving in a clear direction with a clear and manifest purpose. They're often catalysts for positive change.

But before you laud charismatic leaders, give some thought to the drawbacks of being or even having a charismatic leader. They're prone to arrogance and myopia. They tend to dominate corporate identity and make the whole company reliant upon them and them alone. They can become disinterested and unresponsive to others. They tend not to learn from mistakes and consider themselves above others, even the law. Ethical or financial transgressions are common with this type of leader in the corporate world and in the religious world as well. Organizations with rigid structures may not benefit from this kind of leadership.

SOCIAL SKILLS TEST

Take this social skills test to see if you could stand to develop your social skills. Answer on a scale from one (negative, or *no*) to five (positive, or *yes*):

1. I try to see other people's perspectives.
2. In conversation, I sit when the other is sitting and stand when the other is standing.
3. I often do or say things which my co-workers and friends consider inconsiderate or insensitive.
4. I'm told that my behavior is often inappropriate.
5. I rarely think about how others are affected by what I do or say.
6. I always explain all my ideas as clearly as I can.
7. During conversations, people often note how interested I appear.
8. I snap at people in times of stress.
9. Friends and colleagues don't seem to appreciate my unsolicited advice.
10. I don't bother telling my friends how much they mean to me. They already know.
11. I keep up with what's new with my friends, the good and the bad.
12. When I'm criticized, I often get defensive.

13. I withdraw when I don't feel comfortable.

14. I know my friends have faults, but I accept them as they are.

Easy, right? If not, you'll know where you can improve your social skills. Now let's take a look at the impact of leadership in every aspect of your life!

THE IMPACT OF A GREAT LEADERSHIP IN ALL AREAS OF YOUR LIFE

E very year, about 9% of Americans who make New Year's resolutions (about 41%) succeed. But that's still less than 4% of the country's populace who are adept at making goals and achieving them. Are you in that exclusive group? If not, wouldn't you like to be? Read on and let's make that happen.

As we've seen, the layers of your life overlap, and things you do in one area interconnect with another thing in the same area, same things in different areas, and different things in different areas. So, we've broken them up into categories to keep things organized.

The first category is health. Being a better leader means being a strong leader, and strength comes from good health. We've discussed the so-called smart foods and touched on the benefits of exercise, stretching, and sound sleeping habits. But physical health is predicated on sound mental and spiritual health as well.

A few tips and tricks to better health include doing yoga, running or walking daily, a weekly cleanse, and a home workout regimen.

A big part of health is sound spirituality. Spirituality or religion has proven ties to a positive outlook and, ultimately, a longer life. It doesn't really matter what religion or philosophy you adopt. A lot of people adopt several different or even divergent religions or philosophies over their lifetimes, and there's nothing wrong with that. It's a sign of a growth mindset, and we've already seen how key that is to so many facets of a happy life.

But spirituality can help us answer the existential questions which so often cause us anxiety. It gives us a sense of self, a perspective of who we are (and who we are not). Someone with a strong spiritual life is less likely to have a God complex, for example.

Spirituality will give you good sense of the difference between happiness and pleasure. Happiness is a long-term concept, usually related to accomplishing worthwhile goals. Happiness supports self-confidence. Your family and home and career may give you happiness. Pleasure is related to short-term rewards, like an orgasm.

If you're developing your spirituality, try these handy techniques. You can start immediately, if you wish (but read the techniques first, of course).

You might try meditating every morning, just after you wake up. Do it again before you go to bed. Just for five minutes per session. I'll bet you'll find that you're more spiritually attuned, your mind and heart and other chakras open. You may even think about joining a meditation circle or yoga meditation class.

Fashion a strong definition for spirituality and keep it in mind. You might have heard someone describe themselves spiritual but not religious. Do they even know what that means? You should.

Keep a spiritual journal of what spiritual thoughts you have, when and where and why. That will draw your attention to those things when they recur and you'll be more mindful of them. Mindfulness and gratitude are also key areas for developing your spirituality.

Environment is key to developing spirituality, as it is in so many things. Environment both mirrors and affects our daily lives. A cluttered or stressful environment creates a cluttered and stressful life. You may want to include some religious or spiritual iconography in your environment, including crosses, pictures of the Buddha, whatever is in line with your spiritual leanings.

You may also consider decluttering and deep-cleaning. That's good for the body and the mind and for the property too. Redecorating can bring a sense of a fresh start and open your creative mind as well. This includes new furniture if you can manage that. New clothes may be a good way to change your most immediate environment. Replace those tight-fitting clothes with something more relaxed and comfortable.

Romance is another big part of most people's lives, and strong leadership is crucial to a happy and healthy romantic life. Critical thinking will help you decide who is worth pursuing and who isn't. Foresight will help you visualize what that coupling might be like. Reflection will give you time to reconsider your approach. Charisma will make you more self-confident, and self-confidence will make you more charismatic. Charisma is a hallmark of romance. Of course, awkward people find each other and fall in love all the time, and that's adorable.

Do you approach your romances with integrity, honesty, and clarity? Those are the elements of true leadership, after all. And isn't any romance a team effort? Of course, it is. Can you lead your team to the long-term goal of marriage and family and happiness (if that is your long-term goal)? Are you in control of your emotions? Is your partner? You may know your partner's strengths and weaknesses, but do you know your own? Do you keep a healthy climate when you're together?

Here are a few tips and techniques you may use to create and sustain a healthy romantic relationship!

Date at least once a week. This is as important to romances later in the relationship as it is in the first movement of a relationship. New lovers can hardly make a significant relationship without seeing each other at least once a week. And longtime relationships often need to keep dating just to keep the romance alive in their lives. It's more than reason enough! It's also good for relaxation, reflection, action planning, conferring, and more.

Don't hesitate to confer with a mentor while you're dating or married as well. That's very constructive and it's a technique of a true leader.

Go on a vacation once a year. If you're dating, get away from your home base for a weekend. Or travel abroad. It's a broadening experience for both as individuals and for the couple as a whole. It gives you memories and stories to share with others and will likely give you an added appreciation of one another. If you're in a family situation, take this vacation without the kids. You need time together to keep your romantic feelings strong and healthy. Most of your homelife is dedicated to the kids, so when you're not in the home it's fair to have that time for yourself.

Don't neglect to say, "I love you," and say it every day. That's clear communication, the hallmark of a true leader. Saying things gives them power. It's also supportive of a team mentality and crucial for a healthy romantic climate.

Cleaning the house together is a good way to bond romantically. It's healthy, it's exercise, it's a positive and shared goal which can be broken down into smaller, rewarding milestones. Finding old things may bring nostalgia, a powerful romantic feeling, and these things may bring you back to happier or more loving times, resurrecting old feelings.

And when you're together, on a date or activity, turn your phones off. You should be focusing on each other. And the whole point is to get away from the rest of the world for a brief time, so why bring the outside world with you?

The second big area of your life is the professional category. It includes growth and learning, among other things, all of which benefit from true leadership skills, emotional intelligence, and cognitive ability.

Here are some handy tips to improve your growth and learning skills.

Read more. There's a ton of information out there on just about every subject (we've got lots more books like this one, on subjects like overcoming overthinking and procrastination, effective communications for couples, and more!). Set a goal to read a certain amount every month.

Go to a personal development seminar. There are lots of them and some are quite impactful. Research them online for testimonials and agendas, so you know what you're paying for. Use your critical thinking skills before, during, and after the seminar.

Growth and learning are achieved by accomplishing goals. So set some goals at the beginning of every month and make sure they're achieved by the end of the month.

Develop your communication skills and express yourself more confidently in the workplace. This area of growth will help in every facet of your life. Practice how to express yourself more confidently through your language.

Music is a growth tool, and new music will open up new cultures to you as well as excite your creativity.

Time management is a critical leadership skill in the workplace. Practice it and influence others to do the same for maximum workplace efficiency. Consider a time log for yourself and encourage your team members to keep them too. You may reserve the right to see them from time to time.

Classes, lessons, and degree programs are also great ways to promote growth and learning in the workplace.

School is a part of life where growth and learning are central. Are you retaining what you're learning, or does the information fall out of your head as soon as you take the test? A true leader will retain the information for use in critical thinking later in life. Retention also inspires curiosity, another hallmark of a true leader.

To improve your leadership skills, emotional intelligence, and cognitive skills in an educational environment, consider these elements. First, building sound relationships with teachers and classmates. They're your mentors, supervisors, and fellow team members and also fellow individuals. It's a great way to invite feedback, encourage and support others, and accomplish shared goals. Study groups are a great example of this when put into concrete application. It's one thing to get along, it's another to join forces! School clubs are great to, for the same reasons.

Don't forget to take breaks, it's crucial for your productivity and mental wellbeing. This is something a lot of students forget as they study and cram and complete one project after the next. A student's life is a hectic one, filled with wants, desires, goals, tasks, and distractions. You have to be self-disciplined enough to give yourself some quiet time for reflection and relaxation.

Time management is also crucial for students, for the same reason. It will reduce stress and anxiety and result in more productive and effective performances. Use a schedular like a daily planner to keep your tasks and time well-organized.

If you're not in college yet, keep that in mind as your goal and set milestones toward achieving that goal. Completing classes, scoring good grades, and extra-curricular activities are the milestones which lead to college acceptance, though you'll also want to consider getting grants and scholarships, saving money, getting rid of things you don't need to allow for light travel.

Financial interests are a big part of any professional life, and the skills of a true leader are crucial to successfully managing those interests. Here's some sound advice to consider:

Try to save money for emergencies. This isn't easy, and a frightening number of Americans have no significant savings at all. This won't just happen on its own. Set a schedule of how much to save monthly, set up a special savings account, make sure you don't withdraw from it or change the deposit amounts. Make a plan and stick to it.

Debts, especially credit card debts, are a real drain. A true leader knows that interest rates keep credit card debt lingering for years, and this can cause stress, anxiety, and hamper other efforts. Bad credit is also a source of stress and anxiety and drastically reduces anyone's chance of success as a true leader.

Jobs are hard to find, but look for one that will pay your way. There are service jobs open to students, and afterward there are sales and management positions, work in engineering. Don't earn your bachelor's degree and then go be an actor, unless that's paying your bills.

The mentorship of a financial advisor is going to be very beneficial to you later, and it's another hallmark of true leadership. An advisor will help you achieve and maintain a positive net worth, and that's not as easy as it seems. Your student loan has probably already put you in the red, as they say.

Analyze and understand your income and outgoings. Watch these things closely. It's not enough just to spend as little as possible while saving whatever you can. Mindfulness and a specific plan are the ways to successfully manage your finances like a true leader.

Manage cash flow with detailed budgeting based on your income and outgo.

Accrue capital, which is the money left over after cash flow.

Keep family security a priority. This the source of a lot of unexpected expense and those are necessary expenses too. Insurance is requisite to maintaining family security, including medical, auto, homeowners, and life insurance policies. Family security requires virtually all of them.

Investing is a pillar of financial management. Stocks, bonds and precious metals are popular ways to invest, each with its strong points and downfalls. Stocks are easy to buy and sell, but volatile. Bonds are stable but don't do much to increase capital. Precious metals are costly to buy and store and can be unstable. Digital currencies like Bitcoin are popular investments these days. A home is generally the biggest investment a person will ever make, but some question the value of home ownership. There are large associated costs (fees, insurance, maintenance), it's a hard commodity to liquidate and is largely non-liquid. A house pays no dividends and is subject to the fluxes in the market. However, a house can be refinanced and is a sound asset, which is also important to good financial planning. Cars and boats are also assets, as are life insurance policies.

The true leader keeps a standard of living in mind when financial planning. This is associated with income and outgo and budgeting, but it has to do with doing more than saving every penny. It's about making the most of every penny.

A true leader has a financial understanding of the home and the workplace and makes better decisions based on that information. That includes tracing project budgets, the company's annual performance, monitoring or completing and filing household tax returns, and so on. A financial plan for both is recommended to asses and prepare for long-term goals.

In the workplace, teamwork and true leadership are essential. Here's a good exercise to promote teamwork, self-awareness, and other elements of a healthy workplace. Call your team together and give each a piece of paper. Have them write their greatest strength within the team at the top of the piece of paper. Keep in mind that a good team is comprised of different talents which serve different purposes. One person may write *analytical* on their piece of paper, for example.

Now tape these pieces of paper to the backs of the team members who filled them out. Then have the other team members write things which express or explain the person's proclaimed characteristic. The person who wrote analytical may find that others have added detail-oriented or thoughtful or reflects a lot. Those are all behaviors associated with the characteristic of behind analytical.

It's a good team exercise, it provides some objectivity, it inspires empathy as it encourages you to consider other people's perspectives. It supports a sense of self and a sense of acceptance. Try it!

The third significant area of your life is the personal and it includes family and friends.

A true leader maintains strong relationships with family and friends. First, let's consider the similarities between being a true leader at home and being a true leader at the workplace. We've touched on this, but let's put a finer point on it here. The parallels between leading a workplace team and a family (also a team) are striking, and they require virtually the same skillset.

Discipline is crucial to running both a work team and a family properly. Not that this should be an authoritarian approach, though it may be. Remember that different situations may require different leadership styles. And there'll be times in each where a democratic approach is best, sometimes when laissez-faire is the wiser approach in each arena. But you don't want to let either your team members or your children misbehave without being disciplined. Corrections should come with explanation, clarity, and empathy, but rules must be enforced. In each instance, this may mean dress codes and codes of acceptable conduct and language.

Accountability is also central to both workplace and family. Punctuality, deadlines, behavior; all things for which anybody in the workplace or home should be held accountable. That goes for the leader too.

Praise is invaluable in both areas as well, for your team members, coworkers, supervisors, spouses, and children. It's supportive, empathetic, encourages open communication, shows emotional intelligence, and has many more benefits.

Respect is also crucial to running a family or a workplace. Authorities must be respected, but they must respect the humanity of those under them. Deadlines and protocols must be respected, whether that's at the conference table or the dinner table. Respect your co-workers and respect your spouse. Even if you don't harbor respect, it's critical that you show respect. Being outwardly disrespectful to anyone is a sign of lack of self-discipline and is a trait of a leader in name only, not a true leader.

Restraint is also key to true leaders and to the teams they lead. Be it a workplace team or a family, emotional outbursts must be curtailed, body language must be well-governed, one must be mindful of their own weaknesses, triggers must be avoided, behavior modified. True leaders teach this by example. Likewise, a lack of restraint will rub off on either team or family and create a host of negative and counter-productive behaviors like bickering, gossip, backstabbing, and resentment.

Vision and strategy are key for successful leadership in the workplace and the home. Know what your goals are and how to achieve them, in the short- and the long-term. Clearly express specific goals and follow timelines in both cases.

Be participative and directive. It's not enough to give directions. As we've seen it's important to work with your team, to be visible and approachable. The same is true for the home. Help your kids with their homework and projects, mentor your spouse or work with him or her in problem-solving. Use critical thinking and other cognitive skills.

Motivation and inspiration are central to both team projects and family matters, so are a positive attitude and flexibility. Both arenas can be chaotic and may need quick thinking and measured response.

The trust you build by being a person of integrity is critical to both family and workplace.

Determination and commitment are common to both the workplace and the home. Both will present challenges, but you can no sooner walk out on your job than you can tell your wife you're going out for cigarettes and never come back. First of all, true leaders shouldn't smoke for all the right reasons; its unhealthy and sets a bad example. But mostly, your team, your clients, your spouse, and your children are relying on you. A true leader holds his or her ground and advances, they do not retreat or abandon the field and desert their troops.

As to your family and friends in particular, ask yourself; are you reaching out to communicate with them? Are you showing empathy to their challenges and difficulties? These days families are more disjointed and desperate than ever, and a concerted effort is required to bridge the gap.

Here are a few tips and tricks to keep the bonds strong between you and your friends and family:

Call them, or visit if you can. Forget texts and email, nothing beats the personal touch in these instances. What, you never call your mother?

Listen actively, show empathy, don't interrupt.

Take extra time with your kids, teach them self-defense skills if you know them, or how to deal with bullies. That's constructive, positive, and will be a bonding experience.

Fun and recreation are big parts of the personal sphere of your life. Yet they're often neglected in most people's lives with all the hard work and efforts to succeed. So, take time to have some fun, to get away from the grind. It's good for your body and your mind and even your soul.

If you're looking for some handy tips and techniques, you've come to the right place. Consider learning a craft; how to paint, work with clay, something fun and tactile. Remember that you don't have to be good at it, certainly not at first. You'll want to develop your skills like all true leaders will, but the most important thing is to enjoy the process and reap the benefits of relaxation, cognitive stimulation, and personal satisfaction.

We've touched on vacations, and it bears repeating here. Vacations are designed to be fun and only fun. You don't have to be productive all the time and shouldn't have to be. Cultures all over the world include vacation time (the United States is one of the few countries which does not mandate paid vacation time). And there's a lot out there to see; the Grand Canyon, New York City, the Amazon rainforest.

Sports are a great way to have fun. It also has a number of other benefits, including improved physical health, improved hand/eye co-ordination, improved teamwork skills, and personal satisfaction. Studies show that children who participate in team sports are more successful as adults.

A random road trip is great for a good time. Spontaneity excites the brain and breaks a rut. It stimulates curiosity, it introduces new people and new things, new ideas and new information to be used later. It's great for reflection and evaluation, all true leadership skills.

Learning to cook is a great way to have fun like a true leader. It's healthier than eating prepared food, it entails focus and attention on new information, retention, analysis, planning. It's creative, requires curiosity, provides immediate gratification, stimulates further growth. It's like painting, but with food!

Community is also a bit part of your personal life. Besides just your family, friends, or partners, you have a whole support network of medical and legal professionals, advisors, service providers, familiar faces, and others who make up your community. It also includes people you don't know, like the children at the local elementary school, the homeless on the streets. A true leader is mindful of his or her community and knows how to maintain a healthy climate and clear communication.

Consider paying for someone's groceries, if you're capable and they're in need. You'll be showing empathy and enjoying the satisfaction of having helped somebody. If a friend is having trouble, help them in the same way. They'll never forget it. And who knows? You may need the same kind of help at some point.

Always bring a gift. It doesn't have to be big or expensive, a bottle of wine or a houseplant, a bouquet of flowers, a CD of music you think they'd enjoy.

Volunteer work is mentioned often in this book, and it's a great way to exercise your true leadership skills as well as your emotional intelligence and cognitive abilities, including critical thinking. It allows you to practice compassion, utilizes analytical skills, physical activity, social interaction, active listening.

It's easy to see how these areas overlap, how skills in one area are useful in another. Life is complex and hectic, but knowing the consistency of these approaches in various parts of your life will make each one less complicated and easier to manage. Mastery of these concepts in one area will help you master them in another. And you'll be a better example to more people, creating healthier climates and more productive teams, in the home or in the workplace.

Now let's take a deeper look at leadership skills in the delicate (and sometimes not so delicate) area of romance.

LEADERSHIP AND ROMANCE

In today's #metoo world, it almost seems offensive to think about leadership in romance. It has echoes of outmoded macho perspectives. And that's reasonable. We don't enter into relationships to lead and we generally are looking for those who are our betters or at least our equals and not some follower. We want to be encouraged as much as we want to encourage. We want to grow as much as help someone else grow. Generally, we seek a strong partner, physically and intellectually, and that is independent of gender. Men are instinctively primed to look for women who can raise strong, healthy and intelligent children, and that takes strong genes and intelligence from both parents. Each needs the other to be capable, with strong cognitive abilities and emotional intelligence. Those things are crucial to a romantic relationship, as we have seen.

Now let's take a serious look at how leadership is involved in relationships, how it can affect them for good or ill, and how to use your leadership skills in the arena of romance.

Remember that a romantic couple is a team, with (hopefully) shared long-term goals, short-term challenges, which may face unexpected difficulties. So, a couple really does need leadership just like any other team does. One key difference is that, in a healthy couple, there's no one clear leader. In a good couple, the couple leads.

Leadership still includes the same things, like attention and evaluation, feedback and brainstorming, planning and taking action and so on. But a good couple do these things together. Both partners are both the leaders and the team.

It's hard to stress this enough. Any couple with a power imbalance will eventually succumb to resentments, rebellions, miscommunication, dishonesty, perhaps cheating. When the power is severely imbalanced, the results can be abuse, depression, substance abuse, premature death, and suicide.

But the secrets to a healthy, happy, and long-lasting relationships are basically the same qualities which make a good leader (or, in this case, a pair of co-leaders).

Some experts disagree that the most important facets of a successful relationship are financial wellbeing, shared values, ethnicity or religion. But good communication skills trump all of those, and that's the bedrock of true leadership.

Of course, gender will have some influence on various facets of any intimate relationship. Experts tell us that, in general, a lot of women enjoy feeling cherished. It makes them feel respected. Men, they find, prefer to be respected, which makes them feel cherished.

Even so, everybody wants to be treated well, and that's what true leadership is all about. It starts with clear communication. Be able to express your needs and wants in a way that is concise and eschews vagueness. Listen actively and show empathy when dating. Be able to evaluate, analyze, and take feedback. Make measured choices in a timely fashion.

One leadership technique that works perfectly for relationship building is to keep a journal. Chronicle your dates, your experiences, see if you can identify patterns in your or your new partner's behavior. How can you keep triggering good behavior and avoid the negative responses? What about them triggers you?

Another critical step is to consider your leadership technique, as we discussed earlier in this book. You can go back and reread that if you like, I'll wait.

Welcome back. Of all the leadership styles, the servant leader is probably best suited to a romance. The leader who seeks to bring out the best in his or her team and project and company is also the partner who wants to bring out the best in his or her partner and relationship and life. This style infers trust and confidence in your partner's abilities, and that will win their trust and inspire their confidence. They'll mirror that behavior and treat you the same way, offering their respect and confidence in you. With this trust, leadership can be shared by two partners equally. It may also be shifted from one partner to the other depending on the situation. Some circumstances may require the strengths or experiences of one partner, other circumstances may require the unique perspective of the other partner. Once again, it's vital to assess your own strengths and acknowledge your weaknesses while acknowledging the strengths of your team member. That's another hallmark of true leadership.

One leadership technique which may not work so well in dating is a time log. Time management is essential for productive workplace management and goal achievement. But relationships can't really be put on a time clock. A good relationship should develop on its own time, in its own way.

Let's take a look at a few myths of romantic timetables.

Never call back the next day. What a terrible rule this is! The idea is that you don't want to come off as needy or clingy. But not calling also sends the message that you're not interested. It's careless of the other person's feelings and focused instead on your own. That kind of selfishness and lack of empathy are leading in name only; that's not true leadership. Waiting is also gamesmanship of the lowest order. If you like the person or had a good time, call them.

Texting may or may not suffice. If you had a fun date and would like to meet up again, a text may suffice. It's considerate of another person's time and attention, after all. If you had sex for the first time, a text may likely come off as cold and dismissive. Remember that texts and emails lack the nuance of the human voice, and that can make all the difference. Speaking is a much clearer form of communication as long as you're direct with what you're saying. Once you've had sex more than once, a cute text or even a sex-text (or *sext*) can be fun and perfectly appropriate.

You Should Have Sex on the Third Date. Here could be some practical wisdom here. If you wait too long to make a move, your partner might get the idea that you're not interested or that you lack self-confidence. This creates awkwardness which shatters charisma, and that may be what attracted your partner in the first place. Since it's the first thing people notice, this is quite likely. And your charisma hinges on a lack of awkwardness. A lack of intimacy can quickly become the elephant in the room, and that elephant may not leave room enough for both partners. One is certain to go.

On the other hand, some people have trust issues or painful pasts which make three dates feel rushed. Enter leadership skills like asking questions without blame or shame or judgment, actively listening, welcoming and offering feedback, noting how you feel, reflecting, deciding on an action plan. It means responding intellectually and not reacting emotionally.

Some people will have post-traumatic stress disorder (PTSD) or psychological blocks which need to be seen to by a trained therapist. You can use your leadership skills here too. Pay attention to the problem, analyze the information, encourage feedback about getting therapy, solve the problems of what type, consult a mentor, and make a plan of action to go into therapy if that's what's required. Either way, leadership skills will see you through to a constructive resolution.

But the fact is that not everybody is going to be ready to fall into bed, for whatever other reasons. If that's the case, leadership skills will be just the right skillset to help. Use them, along with these techniques, to introduce intimacy while still accommodating a hesitant partner.

Take a shower together. Not to have sex, just to stand naked in front of the other. A lot of stifled intimacy results from embarrassment about body shape and size, various imperfections. A person may have body dysmorphia disorder (BDD) or reverse-body dysmorphia, which distorts their vision of their body. A simple, soothing shower reveals all in a comfortable setting (which is also quite sensual). Caress one another, soap each other up. Don't worry about having intercourse (that's a lot harder in a shower than you may have been led to believe).

Because another source of intimate awkwardness is performance anxiety. This can happen to men for any number of reasons, both physiological and psychological. Showering isn't about intercourse, so performance shouldn't be a problem. This is just a physical, intimate introduction to one another. We'll come back to this, but let's move forward to other ways to ease your hesitant partner into deeper intimacy.

Sensual massage, or even a nice deep tissue massage, are great ways to introduce physical intimacy in a measured manner. There are all kinds of physical benefits to massage therapy besides introducing physical intimacy:

- Relieved stress
- Relieved postoperative pain
- Reduced anxiety
- Reduced low-back pain
- Reduced fibromyalgia pain
- Reduced muscle tension
- Enhanced exercise performance
- Relief of tension headaches
- Better sleep
- Eased depression symptoms

- Improved cardiovascular health
- Reduced pain from osteoarthritis
- Decreased stress among cancer patients
- Improved balance in aging adults
- Decreased pain from rheumatoid arthritis
- Help with effects of dementia
- Increased relaxation
- Lowered blood pressure
- Decreased symptoms of Carpal Tunnel Syndrome
- Help with chronic neck pain
- Reduced joint pain
- Decreased frequency of migraines
- Improved quality of life during hospice care
- Reduced nausea due to chemotherapy.

It's also great for that physical intimacy. It gives your partner a feel for your sensitivities, your instincts. It's positive time you're spending together with a shared goal, and may even increase your spiritual senses as well. Also, it feels great. Who doesn't like to give or get a nice massage?

Dirty talk is a powerful technique too. Verbalizing things gives them power, and doing this gives the speaker a certain power as well. It demonstrates interest and confidence and will instill confidence too. It excites the senses and the imagination. It's something only intimates do, and that helps identify your emotions (remember that?) and to express them. And if you want clear and direct communication of your desires and expectations, another leadership hallmark, you won't find much better than dirty talk.

Some people are reticent to try this, and of course it isn't always entirely appropriate. I wouldn't blurt it out at the Thanksgiving table with the family all around you, but you might whisper it in the hallway when nobody else is around!

Try it ... they'll never know!

Flirting is a critical element to dating, and it's something you should keep doing, especially if there are intimacy issues. Body language says more than your words do, after all. Demonstrate your interest instead of just expressing it.

Oddly, a romantic getaway may not be the best choice for an intimate breakthrough. The pressure may be too great, and a person may feel more comfortable on familiar ground.

You may want to take a commanding approach, play the role of an authoritarian leader. Direct your partner to comply to your desires. Or you may insist that your partner do it and then be compliant. Power is a powerful aphrodisiac, after all.

Meditating together is a good way to relax and reduce anxiety, and it will have all the mental and physical benefits. If you choose the other person as the focal point, that will utilize attention and empathy, two hallmarks of true leadership.

Share your fantasies. A lot of sexual awkwardness is born of fetishism. But a lot of people are nervous about sharing this information. It's something only our intimates generally know. But we're more vulnerable with our intimates than with anyone else. This is the person we're naked in front of, this is the measure of ability and worth as a lover and companion. That's a lot of pressure as it is. But if a person is unsure of the acceptability or compatibility of their fetish, they're not likely to express it for fear of being judged and rejected. However, fetishists often require that fetish in order to function sexually. This lack of communication creates presumptions, assumptions, a downward spiral of awkwardness and distance which can destroy a budding romance.

The tragic thing is that most fetishes are fairly common, and a fetish match may appear to be a mismatch if this subject never comes up.

So, don't be afraid to either ask or declare (both true leadership qualities). Be honest, have integrity. Know who you are and be confident in your standards and ethics. If your partner cannot abide your fetish (or the other way around) then there's probably a sexual incompatibility that cannot be overcome. But you can still be friends. It's another instance of your leadership skills of clear communication and self-awareness being invaluable in your romances.

Now let's go back and take a quick look at erectile disfunction disorder. It can be caused by nervousness, and a nice, hot shower can get both partners over that initial hump. But what about the other causes and effects?

Erectile dysfunction (ED), the inability to achieve or maintain an erection, may be caused by a variety of neurological factors, including problems in the endocrine, vascular, and nervous systems.

ED may be symptomatic of aging, but it is not a necessary result of aging. ED is treated at every age.

Certain diseases and conditions which may cause ED include blood vessel and heart disease, type 2 diabetes, atherosclerosis, chronic kidney disease, high blood pressure, Peyronie's disease, multiple sclerosis (MS), prostate cancer and treatment, injury to he spinal cord, bladder, prostate, penis, or pelvis, and bladder surgery.

Some medications may cause ED, including blood pressure medicines, antidepressants, antiandrogens (used in prostate cancer therapy), tranquilizers and prescription sedatives, ulcer medications, and appetite suppressants.

As we touched on, emotional or psychological factors may also be working in conjunction with one of the previous factors and include performance anxiety, depression, anxiety, stress, and sexual guilt.

Certain factors related to health management may also contribute to erectile dysfunction, including alcohol and drug abuse and cigarette smoking, obesity and lack of exercise.

LEADERSHIP AND OTHER SKILLS DURING A BREAKUP

U nfortunately, not every relationship can be saved, and this goes for romantic and professional relationships, social and even familial relationships. You may have to leave your work due to unresolvable conflicts with superiors or supervisors, or you may be faced with losing a valued team member. Romances end, so do marriages and old friendships. Even siblings sometimes must have to part ways for a variety of reasons. It's sad, but it happens.

And when one of these relationships do end, it's vital that you recall everything you've learned here, as almost all of it will be helpful, sometimes even necessary. So, lets take a closer look at how leadership skills, emotional intelligence, cognitive skills, critical thinking, and social skills to get through a breakup with a minimum of upset or inconvenience for any involved party.

Your leadership skills will be central to the peaceful resolution of a breakup of any sort.

For example, patience is a must. If you're breaking up a romance (or on the receiving end) you'll have to be patient. Let the event happen in its own time. Let the person say what they want to say or process what you had to say. In the workplace, social situation, or in the home, that patience will express your legitimate concern for the other person and your vested interest in their wants and desires and goals, which likely do not correlate to yours any longer, for whatever reason. If you're clashing with an adult sibling or spouse, patience is even more important because these people are much closer to you. And there are external ties, such as children or other siblings, which make some kind of long-term communication necessary if not desirable.

Another hallmark of true leadership, empathy, will be well appreciated by the person on the sour end of any breakup or firing. Express your understanding of their feelings, recognize them as important and legitimate. Be careful not to overdo this during a breakup, however, as it can be confusing. Guilt may inspire you to be compassionate, and you should be. But you may also be unwittingly sending mixed signals which will only antagonize emotional feelings of anger and confusion. If you're ending a long-term friendship, it's likely to be a mutual feeling, so less empathy may be required. You may just drift apart and let the friendship end that way, but it's not always possible. Making things complicated are that coworkers can become good friends and good friends can become coworkers. Any number of things can destroy the friendship but leave the work situation intact.

Active listening, key to empathy, will help you get through any breakup situation, professional or romantic. If your boss is letting you go, really pay attention to the explanation. It could be an invaluable chance to see yourself from a more objective point of view, to better understand your shortcomings, ways you can improve your performance in the next job. It could be that you're not cut out for the job you have, and this may be the only way for you to come to understand this. It's the same thing in relationships. If you're getting dumped, you might have done something wrong. A former friend may have insight into changes in your behavior you hadn't noticed. Or you could be perfect. Either way, the other person has a right to be heard.

Reliability is a leadership skill which is central to navigating a breakup. Maintain your integrity even in that stressful time. It's a crisis, and true leaders are reliable in time of crisis. Don't compromise your standards or ethics for any job or intimate partner. It won't work, as you're sure to return to your innate standards and practices. And you'll resent having to change, perhaps changing those things about yourself you liked best. Just because they're traits a boss or coworker or partner doesn't like, doesn't mean other people won't like them. Sometimes incompatibility comes down to different energies which just don't vibe.

Likewise, dependability during a breakup sends the message to your former partner and to others that your integrity is in tact and that you know who you are. Don't prove your boss correct by throwing a tantrum and destroying the office. Don't prove your spouse or partner right by throwing their stuff out onto the lawn. Don't watch your old friends walk away with their heads shaking while you rave in a drunken stupor.

You'll be leaning heavily on another true leadership skill, creativity, during breakups like these too. You'll need to find new ways to get over the hurt, ways to express yourself. You'll need it to find new relationships, better or different jobs. You'll have to find a way of interacting as adult siblings when necessary while still not compromising the other, new ways of communicating which won't trigger emotional reactions.

Positivity during a breakup will make the difference between a healthy climate and a toxic climate during and after the event. Breakups generally happen as the result of negative feelings and energies, after all. It's a rare breakup which begins and ends with smiles and reason and a friendly hug. Otherwise, you're looking at loads of collected negativity. Feelings of rejection, refusal, anger, betrayal, oppression, depression, and others are likely to surface either during or after a breakup. Keeping things positive is always a good idea. Don't be ridiculous about it, of course. You won't say, "We're over … isn't that great?" But you might make suggestions about the positive aspects of the breakup, that it frees up the parties to move on to greener pastures, for instance. The end of the lingering stresses and the prospects of healing are other positive results of a breakup. Also, looking back with gratitude can't hurt.

Effective feedback may not save the professional or personal relationship, but it's information that could prove invaluable later, giving you an opportunity to see things through somebody else's point of view.

Timely communication is a delicate matter during and after breakups. If you have to break up, do it quickly or they may resent the delay. Don't do it at a family event, but there's little need to wait out the holidays either, as they will only ring false after the breakup and those events will seem dishonest. If you have to do it, just get it done with. Forget the so-called *breakup seasons*. It may be smart not to communicate with a lover after a breakup, as this may impede healing and create false hopes of a reunion. In the workplace, if a team member has to be let go, do it without delay. They may be missing opportunities while you wait to pull the trigger. If an old friend is no longer fitting into your social circle, bring it up sooner rather than later. The problem is only likely to get worse. If this is a divorce or a family feud, there likewise won't be much benefit to waiting. If you're ready to end a relationship, it's probably because you've been waiting long enough.

Team building seems like one leadership skill that wouldn't apply to a breakup, but think again! A loss of a workplace team member will require a replacement, and the team will have to be rebuilt. Other team members may have to be calmed or reevaluated. Keep the team strong despite the breakup by using your team building skills. This is especially crucial dealing with divorce when children are involved. The kids still need their parents, so the team still has to be kept together despite the drastic change in living arrangements. This is a very trying time for everyone involved, but it is especially tough on children. Introducing new spouses also entails team building, and of a most sensitive kind. Here some members of the team (the children, in general) will not necessarily be willing to participate. They'll need all of your empathy, self-awareness, flexibility, and other leadership skills, particularly your team building skills. Losing your friends will require you to build a new team of friends too!

Flexibility is a crucial leadership skill too, especially during breakups. You'll want to avoid being flexible in your position. If you've come to this, backing down will not correct the things which inspired the breakup in the first place. And it may only be delaying the inevitable and offering false hope. But consequences may be many and far-reaching and you'll need to be flexible about how to deal with them. In a romantic breakup, there could be mutual friends involved. Divorcing parents will have property and custody issues to deal with.

Risk-taking is inherent in any breakup, during and after. Just breaking up with somebody is a risk. Will you be able to find another job or a better companion? If I stay, what will I be missing out on? If I walk out on this old friend, what will he or she resort to? If you can't handle risk, breakups of any sort could be torturous for you.

Breakups will also test your abilities to teach and to mentor. How will you teach your children that family is the most important thing if you won't talk to your own brother or sister, or if you're also trying to explain to them why Mommy and Daddy can't live together anymore. Divorce makes teaching kids more difficult because they're only in your company for a limited time. But the skills are crucial to navigate your children through the complexities of a divorce or separation. Chances are your ex-romantic partner or friend or team member won't have much time or interest in your mentoring at that point. But if you are the one being let go or cut loose; the lessons you learn could help you mentor others. It could and it should.

The skills of emotional intelligence will also be invaluable in navigating a breakup of just about any sort, some more than others.

Self-awareness is central to any aspect of anyone's happier and better life, almost nowhere and at no other time than during or after a breakup. If you're being fired, its your responsibility to know why, to know what you've done to warrant firing. It's your legal right in many cases. And it can only aid in developing your self-awareness. In looking for a new job, knowing your skills and weaknesses will help you chose a different career path, if that's what is necessary. If you're losing old friendships, you owe it to yourself to understand both them and yourself. Some cases of feuds between parents and their adult children or between adult siblings often comes down to a certain incompatibility, and understanding that can help us better understand each other and ourselves.

Self-regulation is also crucial during the breakup period and afterward. Not only do you want to regulate your behavior during a firing or other parting of ways, it's just as important after the fact. The days, weeks, months, even years after a breakup can be devastating and inspire feelings of uselessness, helplessness, depression, substance abuse, mental and physical ill-health, premature death, even suicide. A quick recovery for all involved is often the best way, but that required regulating one's thoughts and behaviors. Overthinking and negative self-talk are to be avoided at all costs. Positive activities and energies must consciously replace the negative. If you lost a job, don't languish in unemployment and the downward spiral that creates. If you've had to abandon an old friendship, make a new one.

Social skills will be essential to navigate a personal, professional, or familial breakup. You'll need to show respect, to observe protocols, not undercut the other with their friends. More on this below.

Empathy is one of those skills common to the different skill sets of true leadership, emotional intelligence, and social skills. It's crucial during and after a breakup, though as we said it should be delivered in moderation under these circumstances.

Motivation will really come into play during breakups of all sorts. Professionally, you'll want to send your former team member off with eyes toward a better future, not feeling crushed and desperate. It's part of keeping things positive, one of the leadership skills we discussed above.

Cognitive abilities are also invaluable when navigating just about any kind of breakup and the period which follows.

Sustained attention will keep you focused on the task at hand; retiring one person and finding another, managing what remains of your team, a long-haul project which will have lots of milestones. This is true for social, professional, and intimate relationships.

And because there will be a variety of complex elements to any breakup, selective attention is also crucial. You'll have to pay attention to their feelings and your own, their beliefs and perspectives and your own, other complexities of life. You'll have to stay focused in either a professional or personal arena.

And you'll have to give all these things your divided attention as well. If you're divorcing parents, you have to give the kids your attention, and your spouse, and your job, and your friends. You'll have to use other leadership skills like prioritizing in order to see to all the little crises which are likely to arise.

Long-term memory will be important too. If you're losing a team member, you'll want to use that long-term memory to present a pattern of poor or negative behavior. If you're cutting an old friend lose, your long-term memory of their extended bad behavior will give you cause. It's the same for an intimate partner. This skill will remind you of why you're doing what you're doing even when presented with possibly desperate arguments to the contrary. Long-term memory is what gives you true perspective and it's crucial to your cognitive ability skillset.

Short-term or working memory will be helpful, but it's not crucial to these circumstances. Hey, you can't have everything!

Logic and reasoning, on the other hand, will come into play at virtually every turn of any sort of breakup. You have to stay logical and unemotional. Breakups are often intellectually based. It's usually the result of deliberation, consideration, reflection, and those are intellectual pursuits. By the time the person doing the firing or the breaking up is ready to do it, there's less emotion for them. The person on the receiving end, it's a different story. Without having time to intellectually process their emotions, the emotions are likely to rise to the fore. The emotive side of the brain is the faster to act, after all. So, you can use this cognitive skill to counter emotion, lean toward your better self and keep emotions out of the picture. Emotion and reason cannot co-exist in the same psyche at the same time, remember. Remain reasonable and you can't become emotional. Remain emotional and you can't be reasonable. This principle holds true no matter what kind of breakup we're applying it to.

Auditory processing should be constant. Actively listen, attention and retention and recall. Note changes in vocal tone, speed of delivery, the manner and the matter of what is being said, the subtext (or what isn't being said but is nevertheless true). Never stop listening during a breakup or after, when you're seeking feedback and conference with mentors.

It's the same thing with visual processing. Never do anything without it, especially not during any kind of breakup. Pay attention to little visual cues, body language, turns of a facial expression which reveal what the person you're talking to is really thinking despite what they might be saying. Watch your own auditory and visual signals too, you may learn more about yourself than you care to know!

Processing speed is the last cognitive ability you'll use to navigate a breakup. This is especially true in the period immediately after the breakup. Process the painful information, make whatever adjustments your analysis and reflection and feedback suggest, make a plan and then put it into action. Get a new job, find a new partner, find new friends, change your behavior, move to South America. But it's very important not to languish, to overthink, to get locked into the infamous *analysis paralysis* which prevents further action in favor of constant deliberation.

We move on then, to critical thinking and its applications for a breakup situation, the end of a professional, intimate, familial, or social relationship.

The first element of critical thinking is identification, and you'll lean heavily on this skill. You'll have to identify your emotions at being fired, or you'll be identifying the reasons a person isn't a good fit in your team. You'll be identifying why you want to leave your intimate partner and what you plan to do afterward. If you're the one being left behind, you'll have to identify your emotions and deal with them. You'll have to identify the remedy or remedies as well.

Research is an element of critical thinking you'll find invaluable here. You're doing it right now. But you'll want to ask your mentors how to best get through it based on the particulars of the situation, the behaviors and the personalities involved. This is true no matter what kind of relationship is ending.

Identifying biases is crucial. If you're making your workplace firing based on biases, you're taking a legal risk of a civil lawsuit for discrimination. At best, you're not upholding the best standards, which is what a true leader does. If biases are affecting your romantic life, or your friendships, that's your business legally. There's no law against having biases. And you can't help a bias either. A bias is basically how you feel. Bigotry is essentially how you act based on your biases. So, while you may have biases, you should not ever allow bigoted behavior reflect those biases. That's being a leader in name only, and probably not for long.

Inference will be your best friend in times of a relationship's end. Clear communication will almost certainly be compromised by emotion at some point. People are simply not that forthcoming in such situations (or in any). Politeness and protocol train us not to be completely forthcoming even under the best of circumstances. So, you'll have to do a lot of inferring, no matter what side of any kind of breakup you find yourself on. Be it the true reason for the breakup or the true feeling behind the mask the other wear, you'll do more than your share of inferring during a breakup.

Prioritizing will also be more than handy, but necessary. If you've been fired, you know there's no time to waste. Prioritize getting back on your feet. Did you have to let somebody go? Replacing them with a better team member is your priority and that's easy to see. Heartbroken, abandoned by an old friend? Ask yourself how much that old friend or ex-partner really mattered.

Curiosity is the last element of critical thinking and it must remain alive in your heart and mind during times of a breakup. Be interested in what is coming next. Be interested in what your new team member will bring to the project, or how the climate will be improved. Be curious about your new friends and new partners. You may even want to stay curious about alienated siblings or parents. They're still your family, and a growth-minded person knows that circumstances can change. Just because you can't be in the same room with a person for whatever reason doesn't mean you don't wish them well and want to hear how they are progressing.

Social skills are essentially goal-directed and can vary upon the situation, as we have seen.

Our old friend empathy is central to social skills, because understanding how people feel, being able to share their perspective and even their pains and emotions, is key to social interaction. We've already looked at *The Mighty E* and how it's crucial to our interactions at this stage. Let's move on.

One social skill that will be handy in navigating a breakup of a professional or intimate or social or even a familial relationship; maintaining eye contact. It shows respect, consideration, that you're actively listening. It shows that you're not afraid to reveal yourself, even at that time.

Body language will go far not only during your breakup but afterward. Don't snarl and snap during the unpleasant experience. Afterward, watch your posture and your facial expressions. Don't let the event take over your body. Moving on will mean the self-discipline to control your own movements.

Be mindful (always, but in this case) of being either assertive or aggressive. This is a delicate line that may make all the difference in navigating a breakup of any sort. Assertiveness is about declaring what you want or need. Assertiveness is about standing your ground. Aggressiveness is more about demanding, challenging, attacking. Always favor the former and eschew the latter in any negotiation, be it a contract or a breakup, professional or intimate, social or familial.

Having good social skills includes selecting the best communication channels. Don't break up with somebody via text, don't fire somebody using a bullhorn. Don't end a friendship at the guy or girl's wedding. Don't confront your hostile sibling at your mother's funeral (in that case, you might text … kidding!)

Flexibility and cooperation will be essential in navigating a breakup, especially in the case of co-workers or divorcing parents, as we've seen.

Accepting criticism without defensiveness is another key to handling these situations with skill. You'll wind up getting some criticism somewhere along the line, from a judgmental boss or spiteful team member, from an angry scorned partner or in the form of romantic refusal, from an angry friend or sibling or child or parent. Defensiveness will close your mind when it should be open. It won't be easy, but this is a social skill everybody would benefit from mastering. It's surprising how many people can't handle it even in the most minute increments. The slightest criticism sets some people off into a rage, but these are emotionally ignorant leaders in name only.

Remaining positive is another skill which overlaps from one skillset to the others, but it's a good reminder how important it is in these and other times. In any crisis, positivity is a plus. As are showing respect and being a good learner and teacher. Show respect for the person you're leaving and, even harder, for the person who's leaving you. You may not be able to tolerate your adult sister's company or political views, but you can still retain your good attitude and learn from that experience and share that lesson with others.

Above all, retain your humanity. You're a human being, not a collection of habits and notions. Retaining a sense of your own humanity and the humanity of others will make getting through these trying times easier; professional or personal, intimate or familial. This is the core principle to all the others, the central notion that will guide you in true leadership, emotional intelligence, cognitive skills, critical thinking, and social skills. Respect humanity. After all, it's one thing we all have in common.

CONCLUSION

And that brings us to the end of this particular stage of your life's journey, in search of greater leadership skills. You're now more self-aware of your leadership style, your empathy, and your mindfulness. You're more attuned to your emotional intelligence and have greater control over your behavior and a greater influence over the behavior of others. You've probably sharpened your cognitive abilities, and come to know a little better just what those are. Your new critical thinking skills will serve you in your professional, personal, social and intimate circles, and you'll be able to pass those along to others. That will strengthen your family, your team, and your friendships.

You know how to apply this information to relationships of all sorts and at all stages; at the beginning, the middle, even at the end.

But the journey's not over. Part of being a true leader is to always be curious, always be learning and keeping up with the latest data, techniques, and technology. This book has likely excited you to go on learning in a continuous process of discovery and self-realization. You'll want to take that curiosity and desire for achievement and improvement into other aspects of your life. Better communications in relationships, overcoming overthinking and procrastination and being a more productive worker or manager; there's a lot to learn. We've got the books on these very subjects and many more, delivering the latest information clearly, with practical exercises and just a bit of humor.

Most importantly, you've learned that skills like these can always be learned and improved upon. Your new growth mindset allows you to see life as a process of development. Nobody has to be limited by what seems to be a lack of natural talent. These things are learned, honed, developed, evolved with time and experience. You must have had hope when you started this book, but now you have certainty. And you should have the self-confidence to use this invaluable information to get the job done, for yourself and for those around you. Well done on mastering your leadership skills, now go and master other skills. That is the way to becoming a truly self-actualized person and living a longer, happier, more fulfilling life.

CPSIA information can be obtained
at www.ICGtesting.com
Printed in the USA
BVHW032052230321
603031BV00031B/110

9 781801 342278